Healthcare Massage for Your Partner

Written by Zhang Shulin
Translated by Wu Xuejun, Wang Miao and Xu Hui

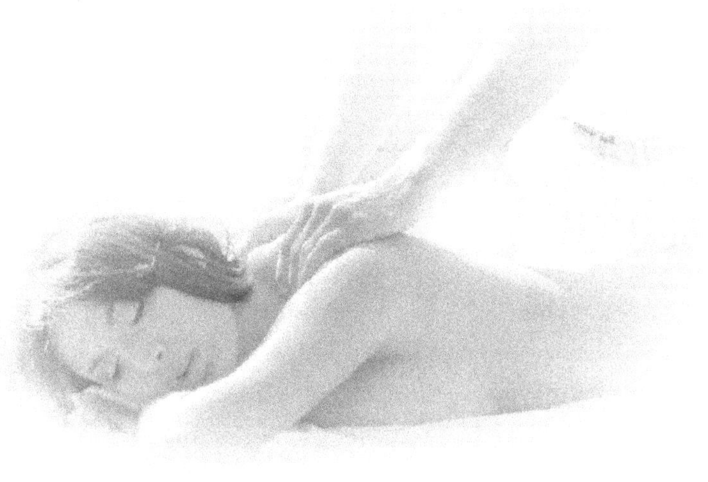

NEW WORLD PRESS

First Edition 2014

Written by Zhang Shulin
Translated by Wu Xuejun, Wang Miao and Xu Hui

ISBN 978-5104-4398-5

Published by
NEW WORLD PRESS
24 Baiwanzhuang Street, Beijing 100037, China

Distributed by
NEW WORLD PRESS
24 Baiwanzhuang Street, Beijing 100037, China
Tel: 86-10-68995968
Fax: 86-10-68998705
Website: www.newworld-press.com
E-mail: frank@nwp.com.cn

Printed in the People's Republic of China

Preface

Massage has a long history in China, it is an important part of Chinese traditional culture. By applying a series of manipulations including pressing, rubbing, pushing, grasping, kneading, foulage, pinching, and lifting, massage aims at soothing muscles, preventing diseases, prolonging life and beautifying the features. Chinese medical massage is acknowledged by people because of its unique effectiveness. As for massage between partners, though not originated in China, its manipulation essence is still within the category.

The massage between partners mentioned here is different from professional massage in hospitals, it is a simplified version for ordinary people. No specific training is required, and it only needs partners' care for each other as well as a general knowledge of massage as introduced in this book. Hence, the techniques don't need to be absolutely accurate, basic manipulation is enough.

As a new health care concept, massage between partners is one of the best ways to ease fatigue, relieve pains and discomfort, adjust minds, improve looks and bring each other closer. It is a flexible and convenient way since the time and location of massage are not limited thanks to the special relation of the partners.

At present, a lot of adults are in the so called “sub-health” state, though not guaranteed to cure the diseases, massage between partners could definitely help to relieve and improve the common pains and discomforts, contributing to correct the body state from being sub-health.

Meanwhile, survey shows that partners who are used to give each other massage are less anxious, violent or hostile, and they are more positive towards life. The caring massage filled with love can bring more delight and enhance the feelings between partners.

Let us bring our beloved ones the most tender and caring comforts through soft massage. Taking half an hour each day for each other can help building up a different and exciting relationship.

Contents

Chapter One

General Knowledge about Partner Massage

✿ What are the benefits of partner massage?

- Effectively relieving common little discomforts to achieve self-treatment and health care;
- Adjusting and improving body functions to timely correct the state of"sub-health";
- Promoting blood circulation to strengthen metabolism and maintain vitality.
- Enhancing endocrine balance to promote excretion of toxins and waste to promote immunity and prevent diseases;
- Relaxing the body to soothe the muscles and alleviate fatigue;
- Improving sleep quality to regain vigor;
- Improving gastrointestinal functions to strengthen appetite;
- Effectively promoting the recovery process of chronic diseases such as strain of lumbar muscles, shoulder periarthritis, leg pain, cervical spondylosis, arthritis, hemiplegia, abnormal leucorrhoea, hyperplasia of mammary glands, prostatitis, and also contribute to the rehabilitation for patients after surgeries and radiation;
- Partners can give each other massage on some sensitive parts such as breasts and the perineal region, and they can also help with the treatment on some andrological and gynecological diseases including impotence, prospermia, sexual apathy, and vaginal spasms, so as to strengthen the reproductive and sexual functions

as well as increase feelings towards each other.

- Local massage can help you to get rid of excess fat so as to keep fit. Meanwhile, it can assist to drain the wastes of the skin to enhance the vitality and skin elasticity.
- To bring more pleasure and comfort to your sex life (Fig. 1-1).

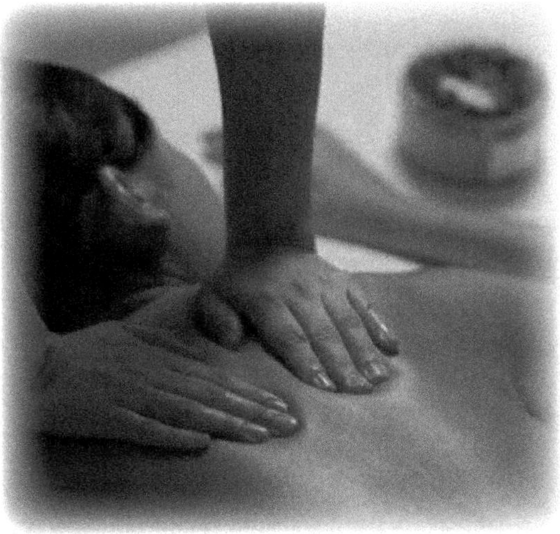

Fig. 1-1

When Is not a good time?

- When there are open soft tissue damages;
- When there are infectious diseases, such as bone tuberculosis, erysipelas, osteomyelitis, suppurative arthritis;
- When there are some contagious diseases, such as hepatitis and phthisis;
- When suffering from hemorrhagic disorders, such as hematuria, hematuria and traumatic bleeding;
- When there are skin lesions, such as scalds, ulcers, and dermatitis;
- When suffering from a tumor, early stage fracture, or amputation;
- Waist, abdomen and hip of pregnant women;
- Women experiencing menstruation;
- Elderly and weak body, over fatigue, empty of full stomach, hangover, severe heart disease and other critical conditions (Fig. 1-2).

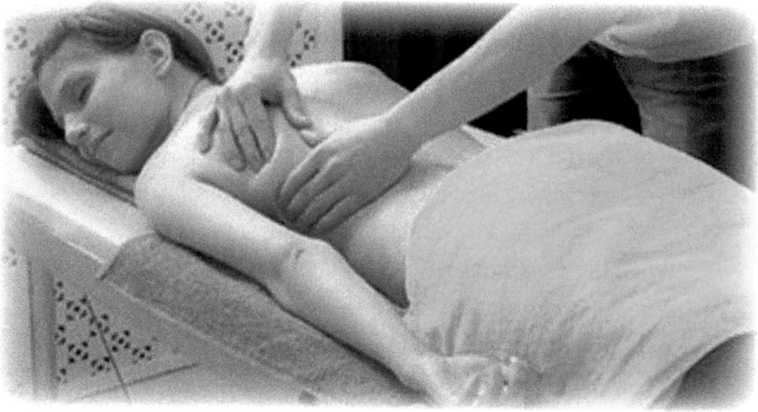

Fig. 1-2

✿ What to prepare?

- When applying massage, the room needs to be warm, quiet and cozy with a comfortable and warm light. You can use the scent of essential oils if you wish.
- You can do the massage on your bed if it is not too soft. Otherwise, you can do it on a mattress or blanket on the floor. Besides, some small pillows are needed in case you need to put them under the head, knees, pelvic bone or ankles during the massage;
- You can prepare a towel to cover the body.
- A little bottle of oil will help the massage. Usually, you can choose

those that would be absorbed slowly such as almond oil, sunflower oil, or coconut oil. When applied in cool weather, you can slightly heat the oil in hot water. It is better to rub the oil on your palm rather than directly drop it onto your partner's body

- Go to the rest room before the massage. Take off jewelries such as rings and bracelets. Your fingernails should not be too long.
- Light soft music can help creating a comfortable atmosphere (Fig. 1-3).

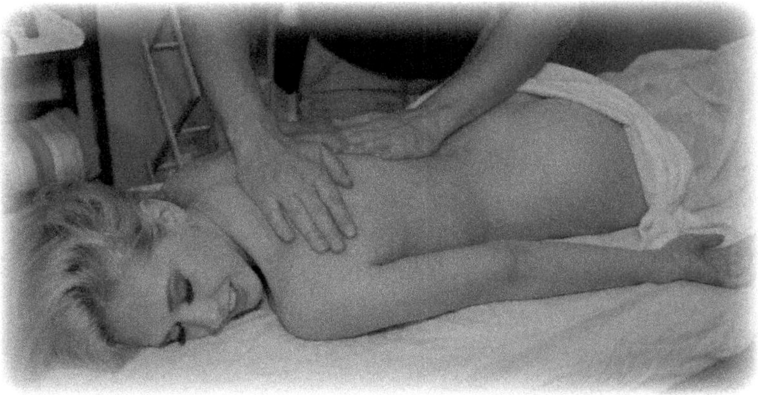

Fig. 1-3

✿ What are the common manipulations?

❶ Long pushing

Technique

Place both hands close to each other on your partner's body and slowly move them forward. Use your palm or palm root to apply stable pressure (Fig. 1-4).

Locations

Body parts with a relatively large area, such as the back, legs or arms.

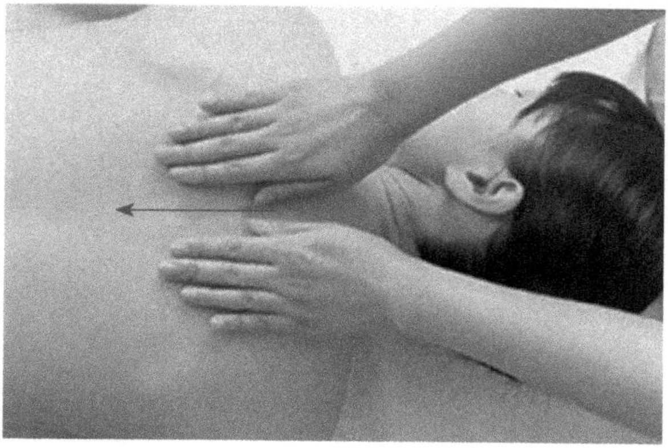

Fig. 1-4

❷ Short pushing

Technique

Alternately and slowly move both hands forward. The moving distance is about the length of two hands(Fig. 1-5).

Locations

Can be applied to strengthen the muscles of smaller body parts, such as calves, thighs and shoulders.

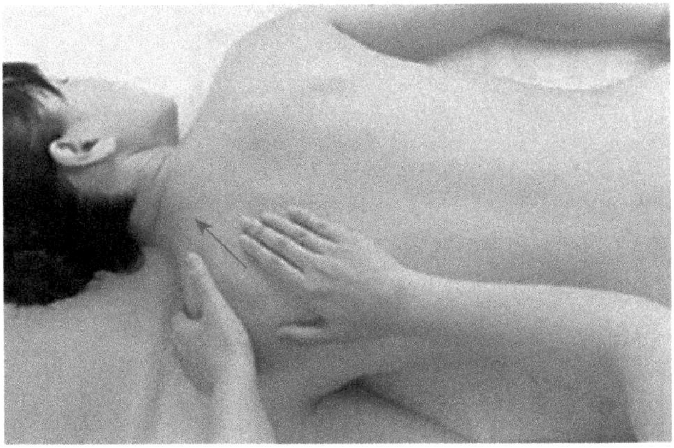

Fig. 1-5

❸ Rowing

Technique

Rowing is actually another long pushing manipulation. Both hands move upward to the top, and then back along the two sides of the body (Fig. 1-6, 1-7, 1-8).

Locations

Suitable for large areas, such as the back and legs. It is often used as a starting or finishing manipulation.

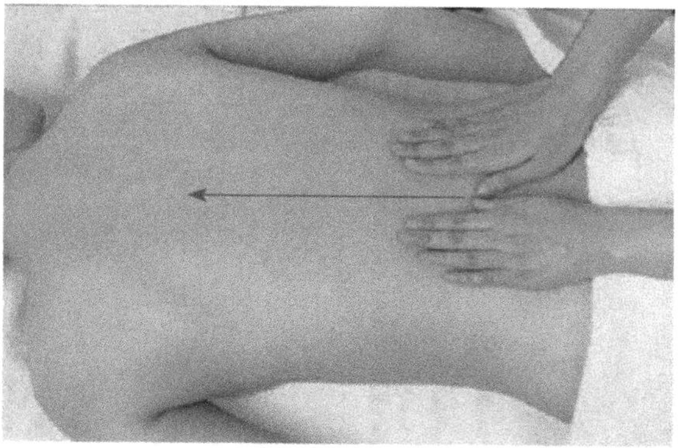

Fig. 1-6 Step one

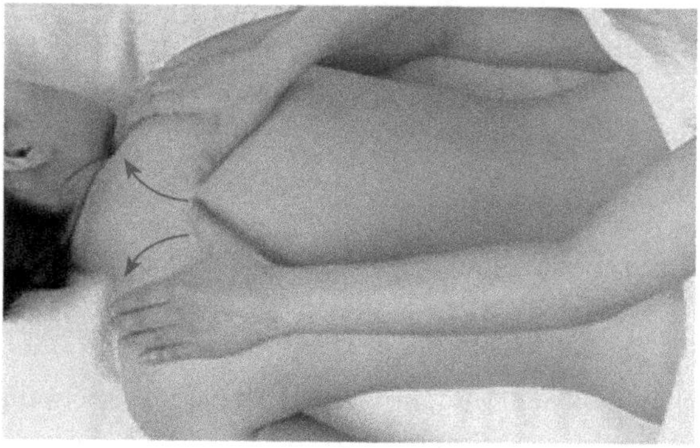

Fig. 1-7 Step two

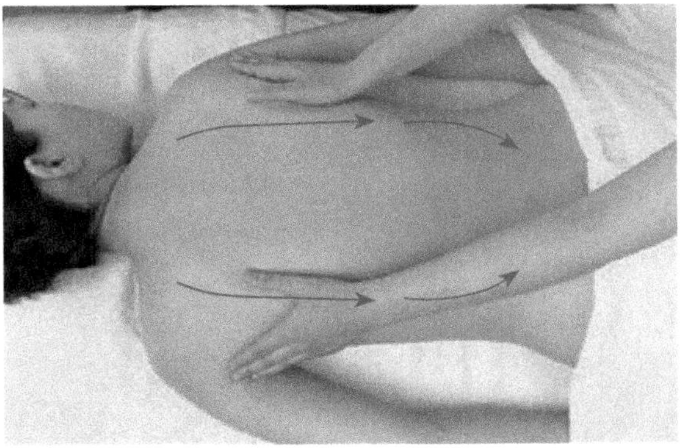

Fig. 1-8 Step three

❹ Finger pressing

Technique

Form a right angle with the thumb and the other four fingers. The thumb applies pressure while the other four fingers keep supporting it (Fig. 1-9).

Locations

Can be used on the two sides of the vertebra, arms, and median lines of the legs. The thumb should press along a line and slowly move upward.

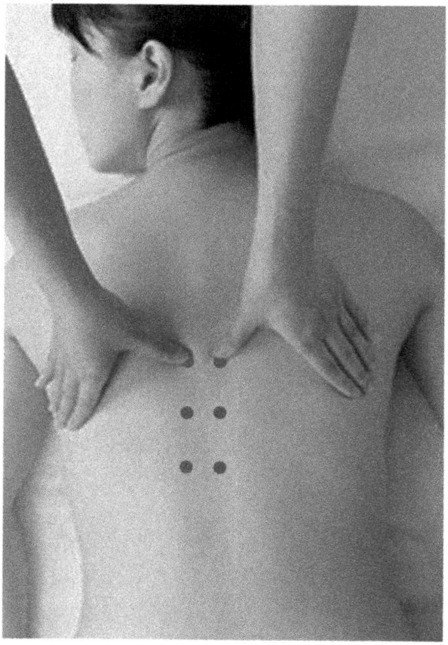

Fig. 1-9 Step three

❺ Soft kneading

Technique

The thumb and the other four fingers hold the body part and knead up and down (Fig. 1-10).

Locations

It can be used on local parts as an auxiliary to manipulations on the whole area. For example, when giving massage on the leg, soft kneading can be applied after the manipulation of rowing so as to further relax the area.

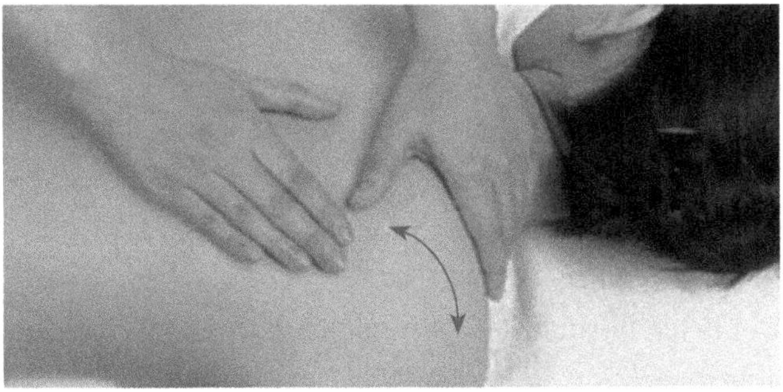

Fig. 1-10 Step three

⑥ Kneading and grasping

Technique

A manipulation similar to kneading and grasping dough using the thumb and the other four fingers (Fig. 1-11).

Locations

Applicable on stiff muscles, most commonly on the limbs and shoulders, use light and slow pressure.

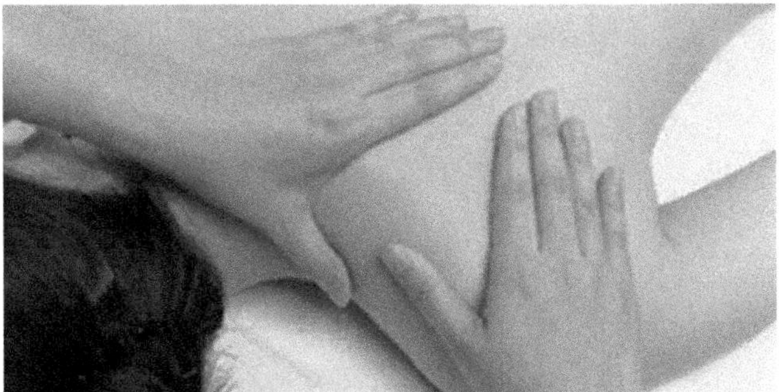

Fig. 1-11

❼ Drawing No. 8

Technique

Push upward in an angle, move back in a round line, then push downward and move back in a round line; just as if you were drawing an "8" on your partner's body (Fig. 1-12).

Locations

Suitable to apply on chest and back, stand on the side of your partner.

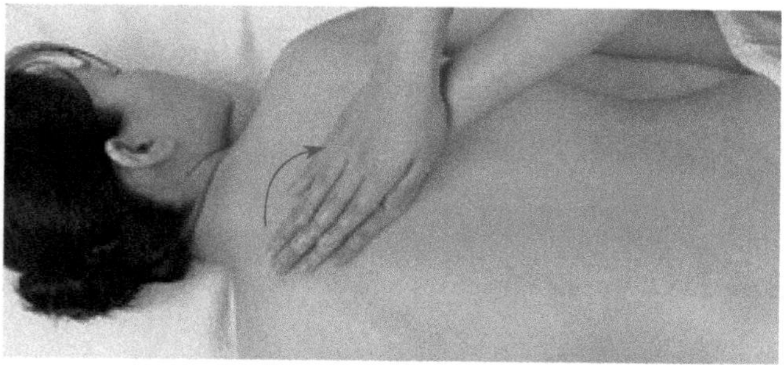

Fig. 1-12

❽ Waving

Technique

Both hands are drawing semicircles from right to left or left to right, constantly moving outwards (Fig. 1-13).

Locations

Suitable when using oil or to calm your partner's mood, can be used on big areas such as calves, thighs and back.

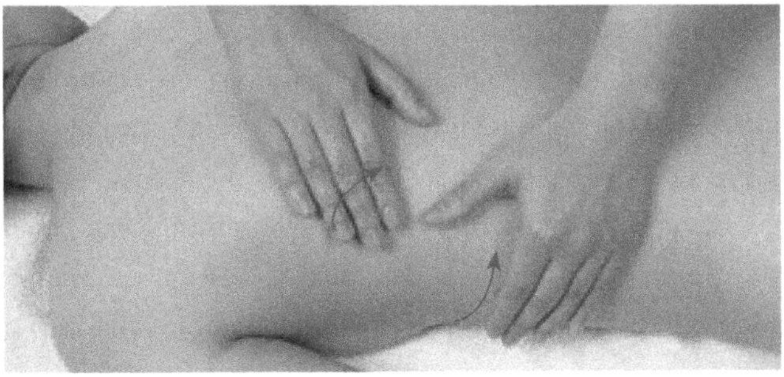

Fig. 1-13

✿ What precautions need to be taken?

The key points of massage can be described with being "enduring, even, forceful, soft and penetrating" which needs to be experienced and accumulated through constant practice.

- The motions of massage should be constant and even, soft and slow, and your hand should never leave your partner's skin.
- During the massage, you can always ask your partner's feelings and needs. Also, when you are enjoying your partner's massage,

tell him or her what you like.

- Power should be gradually increased, too little will fail to stimulate while too much can cause fatigue and damage. In traditional Chinese medicine this is called "Deep but not stagnant, light but not floating". Manipulation can be done heavier on men than on women. Start with light massage, gradually increase strength, and get lighter again towards the end. When massaging acupoints, your partner should get the feeling of "de qi", which can manifest as soreness, or a sinking or expanding feeling, the deeper the better.
- Watch out where you use strength; heavier massage can be applied on the waist, back, hips and lateral sides of the limbs, while it should be lighter on the chest, abdomen and medial sides of the limbs.
- Choose your position according to your partner's position. It should be convenient for massage as well as comfortable for your partner. For instance, when massaging the shoulder, it is better to have your partner seated, while you are standing on the side that you massage.
- Pay attention to the direction of manipulation, meaning towards the heart or away from the heart, clockwise or anticlockwise, to the left or to the right. If the direction is wrong, the massage might not be efficient or it can even worsen the condition.
- When being massaged on sensitive body parts, try to avoid over-cautiousness, laughter and sexual impulses. Enjoy the feeling of comfort and let it spread over your body (Fig. 1-14).

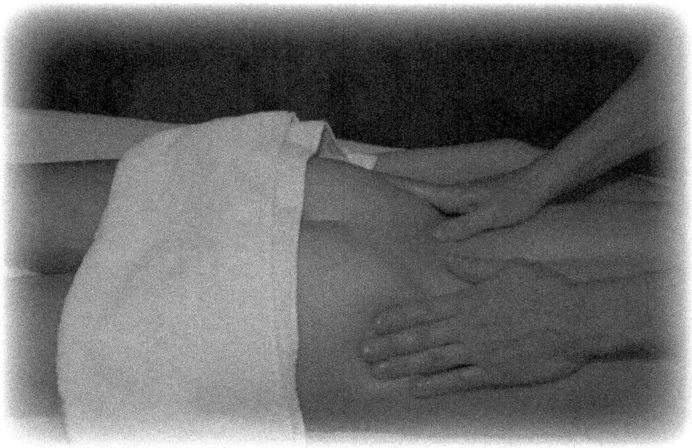

Fig. 1-14

Chapter Two

Become your Partner's Therapist: Massage between Partners to Relieve Common Pains and Discomforts

Cold

Cold is a common disease, any factors that can weaken the defense system of the body or respiratory system, such as catching a cold, being exposed to rain, climate changes or over-fatigue, can cause the rapid reproduction of viruses or bacteria and hence induce its onset. The main symptoms of affect the nose and throat, they include sneezing, a stuffy nose, clear nasal discharge, cough, a dry, itchy or burning throat, or a runny nose. Chinese medicine believes that the etiology of cold is being invaded by wind pathogen. Massage is especially suitable to ease cold since it can clear the heat, dispel the wind, and resolve the exterior.

Instructions

❶ Press and knead Fengchi

Location

Fengchi is located below the occipital bone on the neck, in a depression between sternocleidomastoid and trapezius (Fig. 2-1).

Position

Let your partner lie in prone position or sit on a chair.

Technique

Use your index fingers and/or middle fingers of both hands to press and knead Fengchi using not too heavy strength in a clockwise direction for 60 to 100 times, and then change the direction for another 60 to 100 times. Your partner should get a sore and distending feeling on the acupoint.

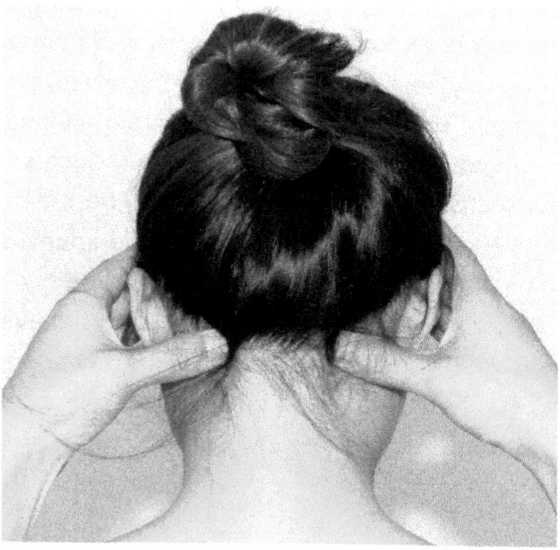

Fig. 2-1

❷ Press and knead Taiyang

Location

Taiyang is located in a depression about 1 finger-width posterior to the lateral end of the eyebrow and the outer canthus (Fig. 2-2).

Position

Let your partner lie on the bed or sit on the chair.

Technique

Use tips of your index fingers or middle fingers of both hands to press and knead Taiyang with appropriate strength for 60 to 100 times.

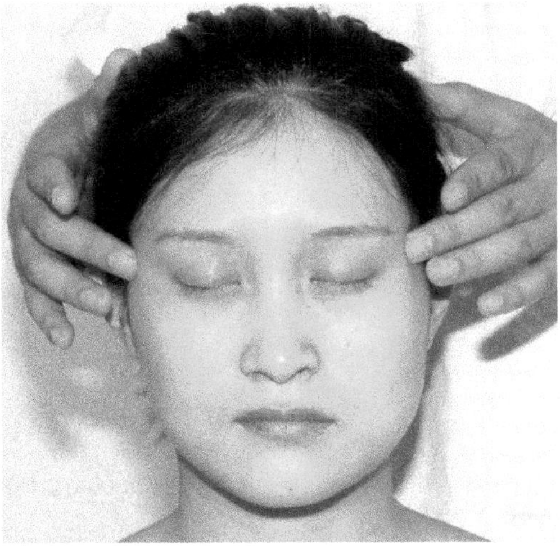

Fig. 2-2

❸ Pinch, press and knead Hegu

Location

Hegu is located on the back of the hand, between the thumb and first finger, halfway down the 2nd metacarpal, at the bulge of the muscle (Fig. 2-3).

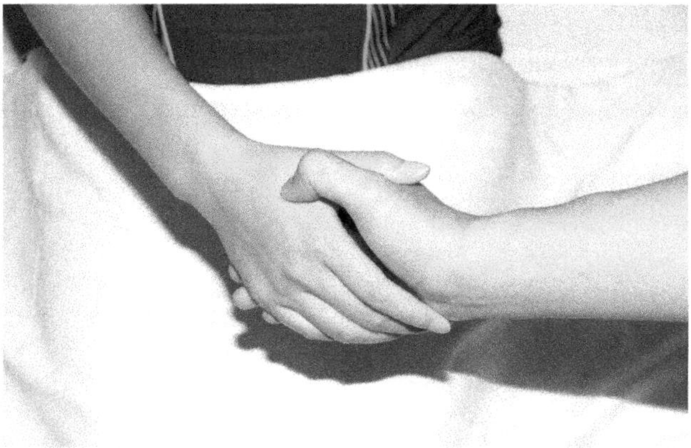

Fig. 2-3

Technique

Let your partner lie on the bed or sit on a chair. Put your left (or right) thumb tip on your partner's Hegu point and apply pinching, pressing and kneading for 60 to 100 times.

❹ Press and knead Yingxiang

Location

Yingxiang is located in the nasolabial fold about 0.5 to 1 centimeter away from the tip of nasal ala(Fig. 2-4).

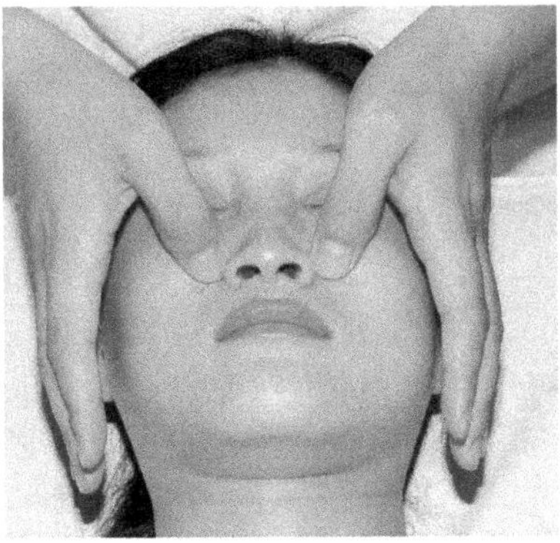

Fig. 2-4

Position

Let your partner lie on the bed or sit on the chair.

Technique

Use the tips of index fingers or middle fingers of both hands to press and knead the Yingxiang points on both sides for 60 to 100 times.

Tips

1. The above acupoints are the main and most effective points to prevent cold.

2. Every massage on the above acupoints can both prevent and treat cold. After the massage, headache can be relieved and a stuffy nose can be improved.

✿ Cold Induced Fever

Most people will get a fever after catching a cold caused by viral infection. According to traditional Chinese medicine, the body's natural response is to fight the pathogen. Massage can disperse the wind, resolve the exterior, clear the head, brighten the eyes and remove the heat.

Instructions

❶ Push and knead Kongzui

Location

When you stretch the forearm with the palm facing upward, Kongzui is located on the medial side of the forearm, at about 4/9 of the line between Taiyuan and Chize(Fig. 2-5).

Position

Let your partner sit on a chair or lie on the bed.

Technique

Put the tip of your thumb opposite to the other four fingers, push and knead the point 36 times.

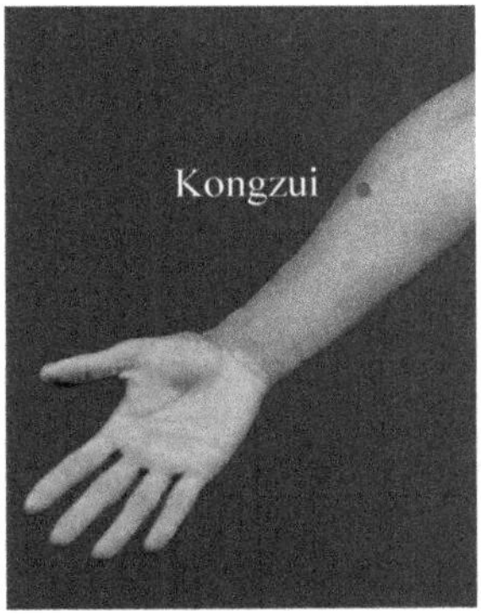

Fig. 2-5

❷ Press and knead Hegu

Location

Hegu is located on the back of the hand, between the thumb and first finger, halfway down the 2nd metacarpal, at the bulge of the muscle (Fig. 2-6).

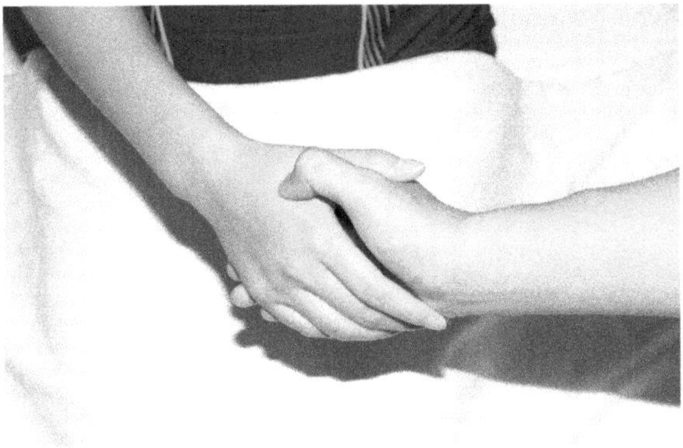

Fig. 2-6

Position

Let your partner sit on the chair or lie on the bed.

Technique

After pressing the Kongzui point, ask your partner to turn the hand. Put your thumb onto Hegu and the other fingertips on the other side of your partner's thumb, so that you can massage Hegu while applying pressure from the other side of it. Repeat 36 times.

Tips

1. Pinching, pressing and kneading on the above two acupoints can treat colds without sweating.

2. The massage should produce a feeling of soreness, distention or tingling.

Cold Induced Stuffy Nose

When catching a cold, the nasal mucosa swells and inflammation can cause it to exsudate, causing a stuffy nose. According to traditional Chinese medicine, a stuffy nose is caused by wind invading the exterior (skin and hair) and interior (lung), resulting in a failure of the lungs' down-bearing action, which leads to an obstruction of the nose. Massage can dispel the wind, resolve the exterior, free the orifices so as to relieve the stuffy nose.

Instructions

❶ Push and knead Dazhui

Location

Let your partner sit tight and lower his/her head. The acupoint of Dazhui is located in the depression below the seventh cervical spinous process (Fig. 2-7).

Position

Let your partner sit on the chair.

Technique

Press the middle finger of your right hand on the Dazhui point, and put the middle finger of your left hand on the other middle finger to knead the point in a clockwise and anticlockwise direction

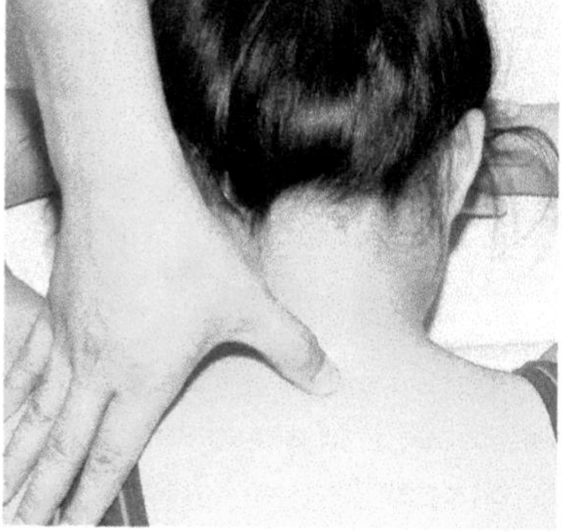

Fig. 2-7

respectively, both for 30 times.

❷ Push and knead Fengchi

Location

Fengchi is located below the occipital bone on the neck, in a depression between sternocleidomastoid and trapezius (Fig. 2-8).

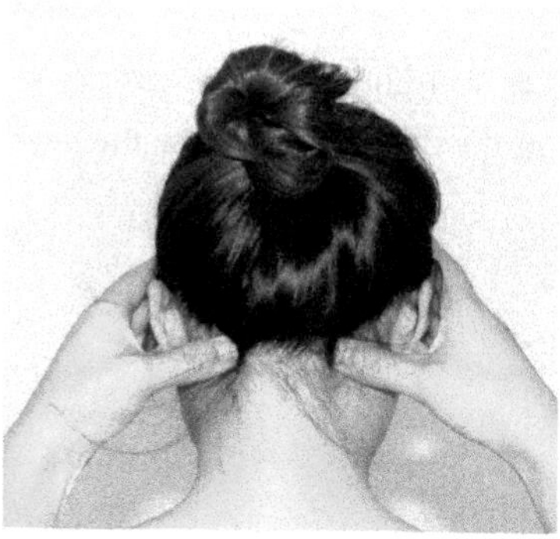

Fig. 2-8

Position

Let your partner lie on the chair.

Technique

Press the point with your right index finger and left index finger respectively, both for 30 times.

❸ Simulate motion of Gaohuang

Location

Gaohuang is located below the fourth thoracic spinous process, in a vertical line with the medial shoulder blade. Your partner will feel soreness (Fig. 2-9).

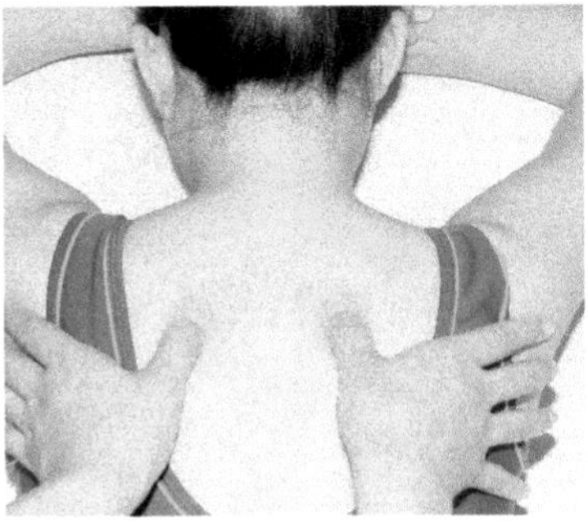

Fig. 2-9

Position

Let your partner lie on his/her stomach.

Technique

Let your partner naturally drop her/his arms, slightly shake the shoulder joints on both sides and promote rotation of the shoulder blade so as to move the Gaohuang point.

❹ Rub Cuanzhu and Yingxiang

Location

Cuanzhu is located in the depression near the medial side the of eyebrow (Fig. 2-10). Yingxiang is located in the nasolabial fold which is 0.5 to 1 centimeter away from the nasal ala (Fig. 2-11).

Position

Let your partner sit on the chair or lie on the bed.

Technique

Use the inside of your middle fingers to rub both sides of your partner's nose from Cuanzhu to Yingxiang, repeat 30 times, and then slightly press and knead the Yingxiang point for 5 to 10 minutes.

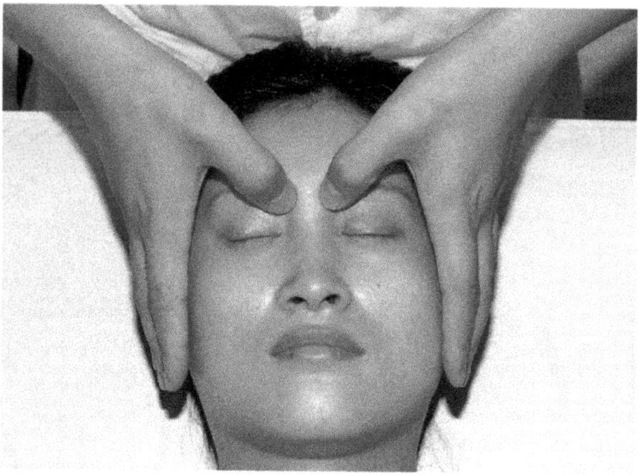

Fig. 2-10

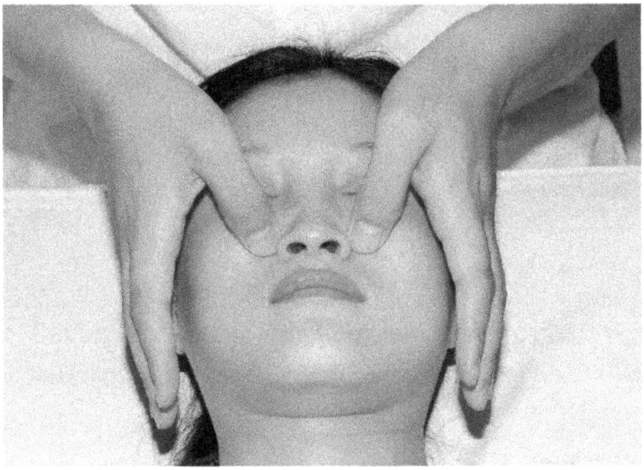

Fig. 2-11

❺ Press and knead Suliao

Location

Suliao is located in the middle of the nose tip(Fig. 2-12).

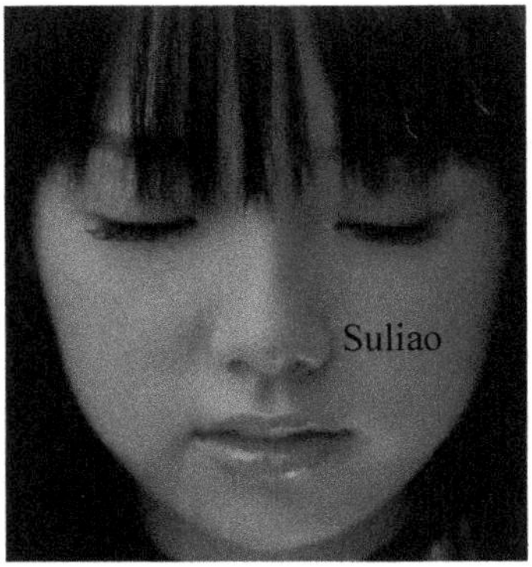

Fig. 2-12

Position

Let your partner lie on the bed or sit on the chair.

Technique

Press and knead Suliao point with the tip of your middle finger.

Tips

1. Try to provoke a feeling of soreness or distention.
2. You can repeat this technique several times a day.

Eyestrain

Eyestrain may be caused by ametropia or eye diseases, but even more by factors as age, constitution, environmental factors, and life style including lack of physical practice, malnutrition, constant insomnia, irregular life, excessive smoking and drinking as well as careless eye hygiene. People above forty start to have aging eyes, if they don't use glasses, they may easily get eyestrain. Lack of light, reading small words, reading too long or working with an unfixed range of vision can strain the eyes and lead to tension. According to traditional Chinese medicine, eyestrain is caused by qi stagnation and blood stasis, deficiency of liver and kidneys, qi and blood deficiency or effulgent fire of the heart and liver. Massage can effectively relieve eyestrain, bring enough rest to the eyes, stimulate the eye muscles which are easily to age, as to let the eyes regain vitality.

Instructions

❶ Press and knead Tianying

Location

Tianying is also called Ashi point, Buding point or point of tenderness; its location and name are changing according to the disease. For this disease, the Tianying point can usually be found below the eyebrow or above the eye socket (Fig 2-13).

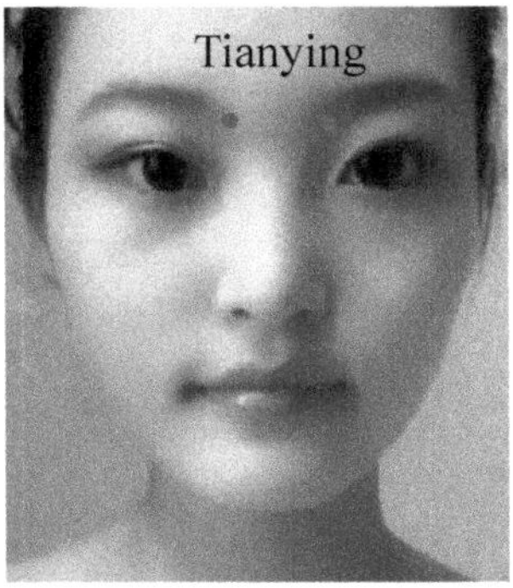

Fig. 2-13

Position

Let your partner sit on the chair or lie on the bed.

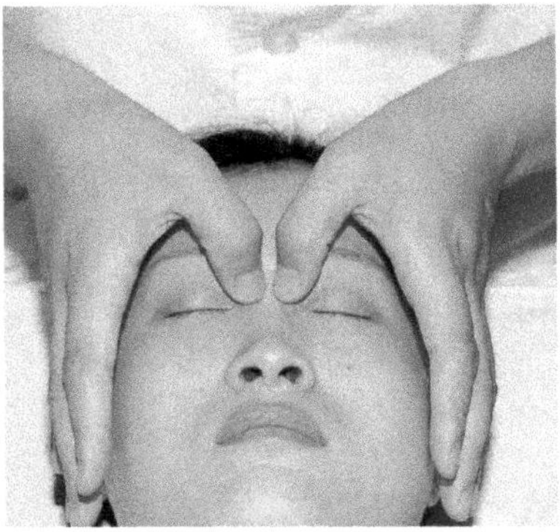

Fig. 2-14

Technique

Press and knead the Tianying point with your thumbs for 5 minutes.

❷ Squeeze and press Jingming

Location

It is located in the depression slightly above the inner canthus (Fig 2-14).

Position

Let your partner sit on the chair or lie on the bed.

Technique

Slightly knead and press Jingming with your thumb, and then squeeze upward.

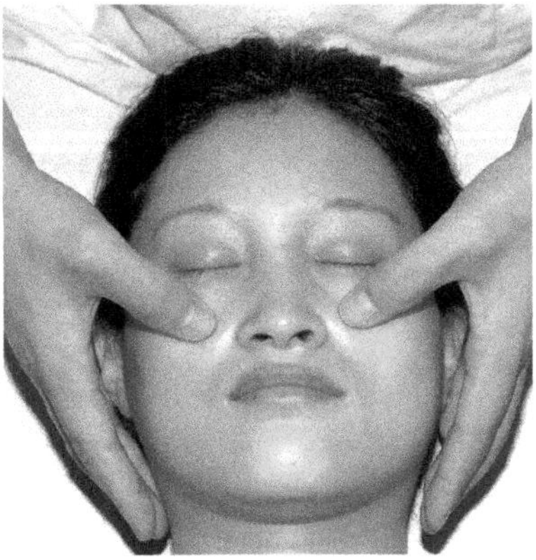

Fig. 2-15

❸ Press and knead Sibai

Location

Let your partner look straight, Sibai is located in the depression below the pupil and above the cheekbone (Fig 2-15).

Position

Let your partner sit on the chair or lie on the bed.

Technique

Knead and press Sibai with your index finger.

❹ Press Taiyang and scrape the rim of the eye

Location

Taiyang is located in a depression about one finger-width posterior to the lateral end of the eyebrow and the outer canthus (Fig 2-16).

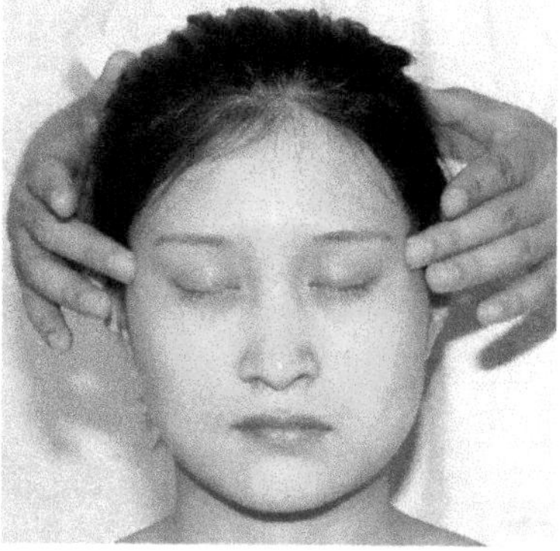

Fig. 2-16

Position

Let your partner sit on the chair or lie on the bed.

Technique

Use your thumb to press Taiyang and the medial side of your index finger's knuckle to scrape along the eye socket, starting on the inside and moving up and out, and then back in a circle. This will stimulate the acupoints around the eye socket: Cuanzhu, Yuyao, Sizhukong, Tongziliao, Qiuhou and Chengqi.

Tips

1. For the best results, you can combine the techniques listed above.

2. Use light strength and slow movements to achieve a feeling of soreness and distention.

Toothache

Toothache is the most common symptom of tooth diseases including dentalcaries, acute pulpitis, chronic pulpitis, paradentitis, and gingivitis. Besides, some neurological diseases such as trigeminal neuralgia and peripheral facial neuritis, and some chronic diseases, such as hypertension leading to dental pulp congestion or diabetes leading to dental pulp blood vessel inflammation and necrosis, may also cause toothache. According to traditional Chinese medicine, toothache can be divided into deficiency and excess types. The excess fire type leads to the most intensive toothaches, the gums are red and swollen, and patients usually don't dare to eat hot things. The deficient fire toothache is less intensive but persistent, the gums are not obviously red and swollen. Massage on several acupoints can help to relieve the pain.

Instructions

❶ Press Hegu

Location

Hegu is located on the back of the hand, between the thumb and first finger, halfway down the 2nd metacarpal, at the bulge of the muscle (Fig 2-17).

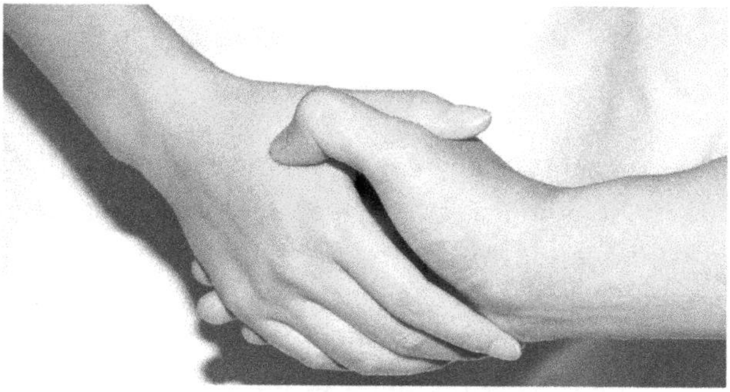

Fig. 2-17

Position

Let your partner to sit on the chair or lie on the bed.

Technique

Use the tip of your thumb to press the point and gradually increase the strength for one to two minutes.

❷ Press Jiache

Location

It is located at about one finger-width from the angle of the jaw, at the highest point of the m. masseter when chewing (Fig 2-18).

Position

Let your partner sit on the chair or lie on the bed.

Technique

Use both thumbs to press the respective Jiache points, gradually increase pressure for one to two minutes. It can resolve tetany, relieve pain, activate blood and disperse swelling.

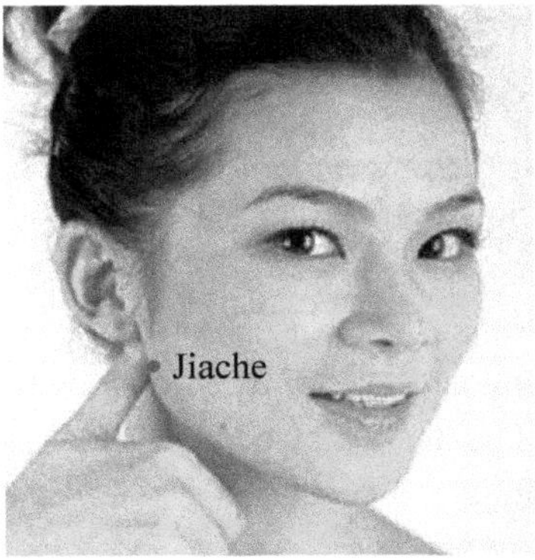

Fig. 2-18

Tips

If you apply the techniques described above 3 to 4 times a day, the symptoms of toothache will be obviously relieved.

✿ Chronic Pharyngitis

The main symptoms of chronic pharyngitis include a dry throat, stabbing pain, pruritis, and foreign body sensation. It is usually aggravated by changes of mood or weather. According to traditional Chinese medicine chronic, pharyngitis is caused by the disharmony of qi, yang, blood and fluids, malnutrition of the throat, qi stagnation and blood stasis. Massage can free the channels, activate blood circulation and transform stasis, eliminate inflammation and resolve swelling so as to satisfactorily treat chronic pharyngitis.

Instructions

❶ Press Lianquan

Location

Lianquan is located on the anterior midline of the throat, in a depression above the hyoid bone (Fig 2-19).

Position

Let your partner sit on the chair or bed.

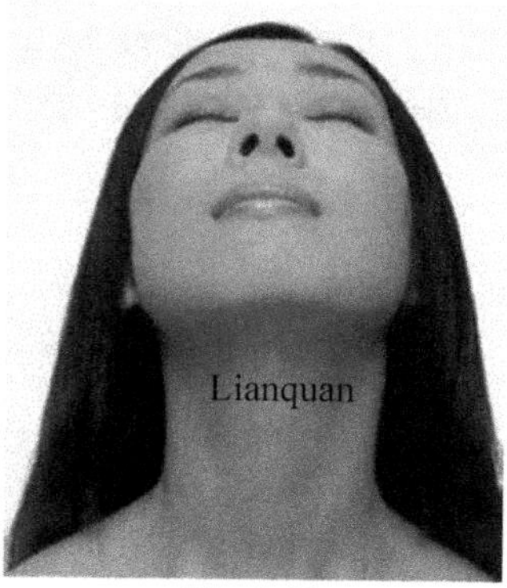

Fig. 2-19

Technique

Sit face to face with your partner and press and knead her/his Lianquan point with your thumb for 100 times.

❷ Press Renying

Location

Renying is located at about two centimeters beside the Adam's apple (Fig 2-20).

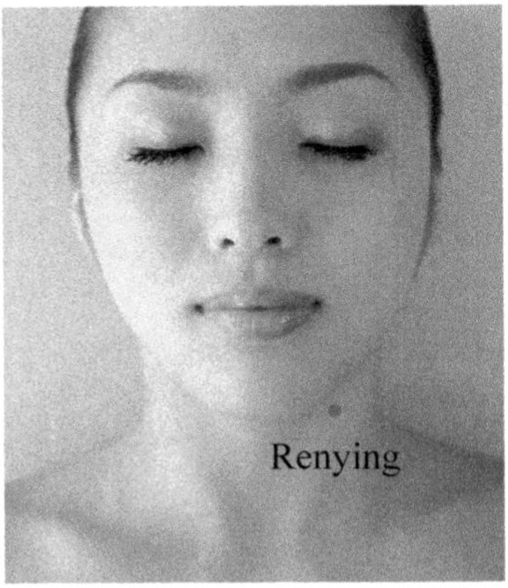

Fig. 2-20

Position

Let your partner sit on the chair or bed.

Technique

Press and knead the Renying points on both sides with your index finger and thumb, repeat 100 times. Try to produce a sensation of soreness and distention.

❸ Grasp thenar, Shaoshang and Hegu

Location

Thenar is the thick muscle at the thumb root (Fig 2-21); Shaoshang is located at the lateral side of the thumb, about 0.3 centimeters from the nail (Fig 2-22). Hegu is located on the back of the hand, between the thumb and first finger, halfway down the 2nd metacarpal, at the bulge of the muscle (Fig 2-23).

Position

Let your partner sit on the chair or bed.

Technique

Grasp hard on thenar, Shangshang and Hegu, 20-30 times respectively.

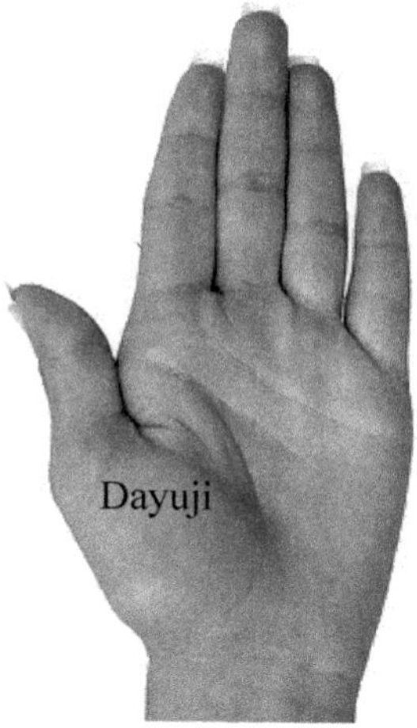

Fig. 2-21

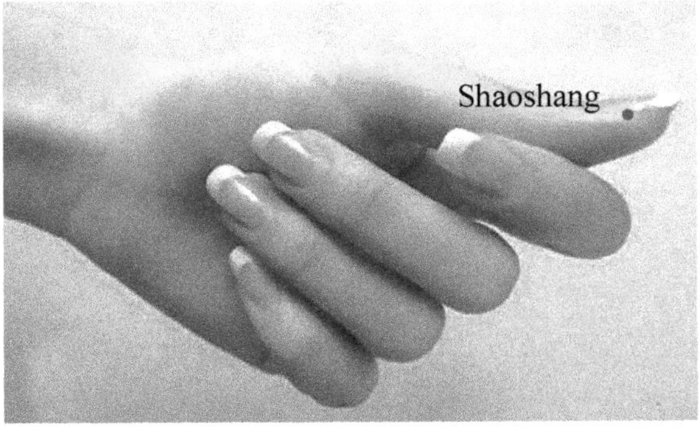

Fig. 2-22

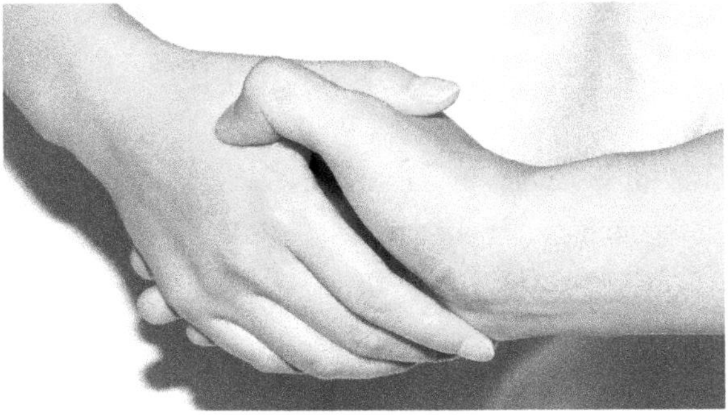
Fig. 2-23

❹ Press and knead Taiyang

Location

Taiyang is located in a depression about one finger-width posterior to the lateral end of the eyebrow and the outer canthus (Fig 2-24).

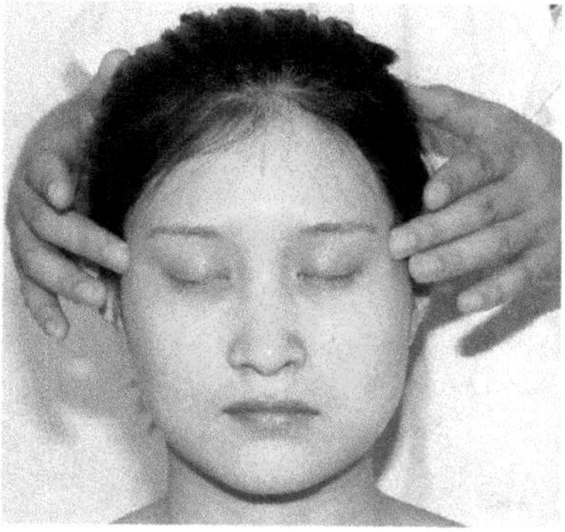

Fig. 2-24

Position

Let your partner sit on the chair or bed.

Technique

Stand or sit behind your partner, and press and knead Taiyang 50 times with the thenars of both hands.

Tips

1. Apply the sequence described above once a day.

2. Use gentle manipulation to achieve a feeling of soreness and distention.

Headache

There are many reasons that can cause headache which can be mainly divided into three types. The most common type of headache is caused by the contraction of muscles of head and neck, brought about by work or family pressure, incorrect walking or sleeping postures or often lowering the head. The second one is migraine, caused by the contraction of blood vessels of the head, it does not last too long and is stress-related. For instance, migraine might occur when coming to a new environment or starting a holiday after completing a tough assignment. The third type of headache is caused by various diseases of the head, eyes, ears or even teeth, which are rare and accompanied by various symptoms.

According to traditional Chinese medicine, wind, cold, damp and heat pathogens can invade the head, as a careless lifestyle can result in the obstruction of qi and blood in the channels, causing headaches. Long-term anxiety and depression causes the liver qi to stagnate, which can also result in headaches. Innate insufficiency, sexual exhaustion hurting the kidneys, damage of yin essence, qi and blood deficiency in aged people or insufficient qi and blood in the brain due to long-term diseases, delivery or loss of blood can all cause headaches. Moreover, an improper diet or overeating can damage the spleen and stomach, leading to poor spleen yang, damp phlegm obstructing the orifices and clear yang failing to support the head, resulting in headaches.

Massage can effectively relieve the headaches and migraine caused by non-organic pathological changes such as cold, heatstroke, neurological diseases or insufficient sleep.

Instructions

❶ Squeeze the muscles of the neck (Ashi points)

Location

The most tender points in the nape area (Fig. 2-25).

Position

Let your partner sit on the chair or bed.

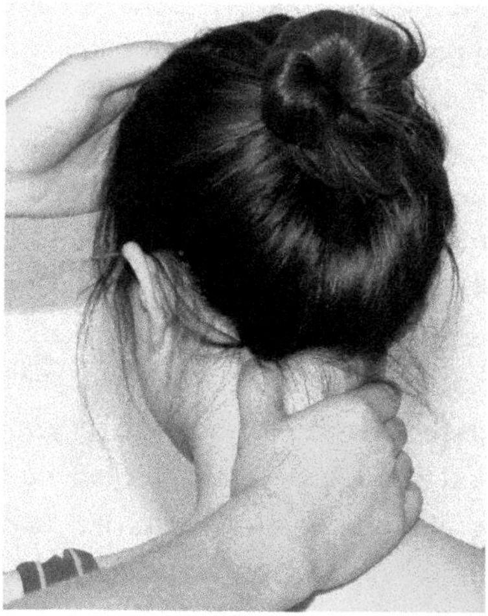

Fig. 2-25

Technique

Squeeze the muscles of the nape area with one hand or both hands, use a rotating manipulation on the painful parts and stretch your partner's head 100 times.

❷ Press the Ashi points under the occiput.

Location

The Ashi points are the tender points under the occiput (Fig. 2-26).

Position

Let your partner sit on the chair or bed.

Technique

Massage the tender points under the occiput, use the thumbs to press the occipital bone tightly and then loosely, repeat until the

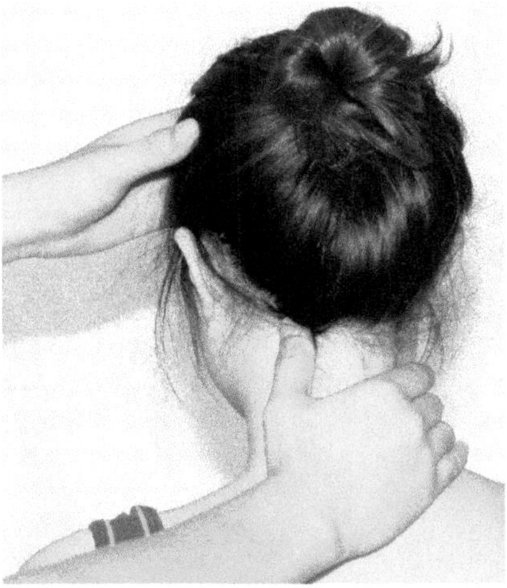

Fig. 2-26

fingers start to feel sore. After a few dozen times the headache should recede, the massage can be repeated after a few hours.

❸ Manipulations on Chize

Location

Ask your partner to sit tight with palms facing upward and the elbows slightly flexed. Chize is located on the elbow. Ask your partner to raise the arm, the point is on the lateral side of the thick sinew in the middle of the medial side of the arm. You can also look for the depression of the radial side of the biceps, where the point is on the transverse elbow striation (Fig. 2-27).

Position

Let your partner sit on the chair or bed.

Technique

Press Chize and the tender area around it until the headache is

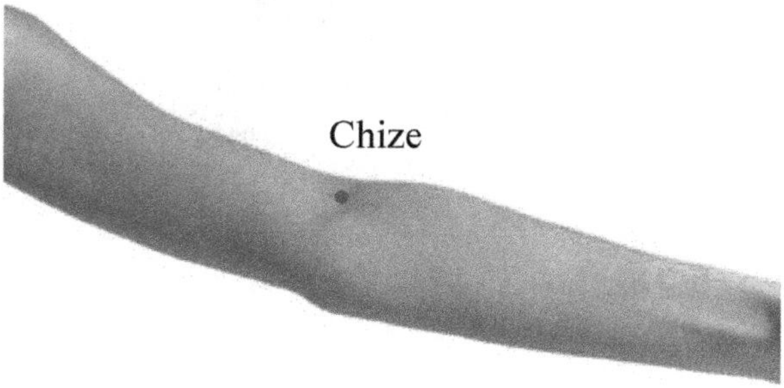

Fig. 2-27

relieved. Your partner should not feel pain at the points.

❹ Manipulations on Tianzhu

Location

Tianzhu is located in a depression at the lateral side of the trapezius, 4.5 centimeters beside the first spinous process (Fig. 2-28).

Position

Let your partner sit on the chair or bed.

Technique

Cross your thumbs and put them on the points on both sides, first press the point on the right side then press the left one. Ask your partner to slightly lean his/her head to the left, breathe out and count to one and two, meanwhile you increase the force; when your partner counts to three, you should keep on pressing the point; when your partner counts to four, five, and six, she/he shall breathe in, relax the body, and lean the head back. Then press the acupoint on the other side with the head leaning to the opposite side.

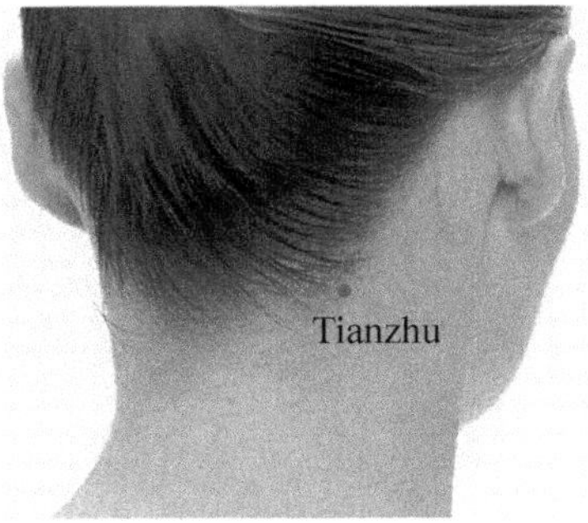

Fig. 2-28

❺ Manipulations on Taichong

Location

Taichong is located in the depression distal to the junction of the first and second metatarsal bones (Fig. 2-29).

Position

Let your partner to sit on the chair or bed.

Technique

Ask your partner to put his/her left foot on the chair, and press the point with the middle finger of your right hand. Ask your partner to breathe out and count to one and two, meanwhile you increase the force; when your partner counts to three, you should hold the pressure on the point; when your partner counts to four, five, and six, she/he shall breathe in and relax the body.

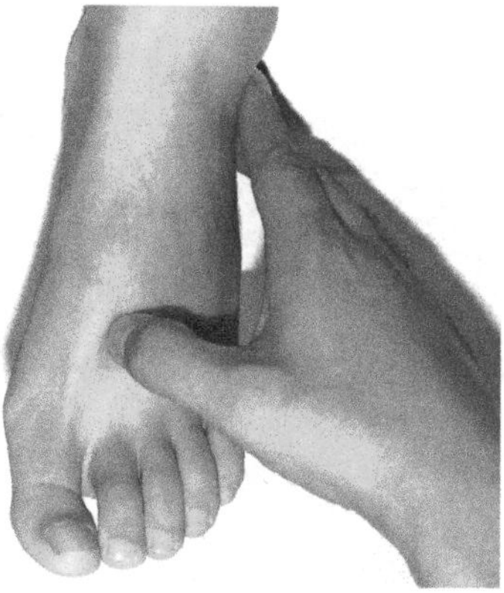

Fig. 2-29

Tips

1. When there is a sudden onset of migraine or headache, please apply the massage on your partner right away, usually an instant effect can be achieved.

2. Every massage can prevent the sudden onset of the disease.

Carsickness

Carsickness generally refers to dizzyness or vomiting when taking cars, boats, or airplanes. The vibration causes the inner ear to fail adjusting the sense of balance and leads to further irritation of the sympathetic nervous system. According to traditional Chinese medicine, carsickness is due to marrow sea deficiency and governor vessel insufficiency. It is usually seen in children as their body's qi is not yet consolidated, in most cases it will disappear when growing up. Carsickness in adults is usually due to inadequate rest, over-eating or a poor adaptive ability to vehicles. Massage can quiet the heart and spirit, resolve depression, loosen the chest, regulate qi, downbear counterflow and stop vomiting.

Instructions

❶ Pressing Neiguan

Location

Let your partner stretch his/her arm with the palm facing up. The location of Neiguan is 6.5 centimeters above the wrist transverse striation, between two sinews (Fig. 2-30).

Position

Let your partner sit on the chair or bed.

Technique

Use some force to press Neiguan with your thumb for one to five minutes. This is the most common way to treat carsickness.

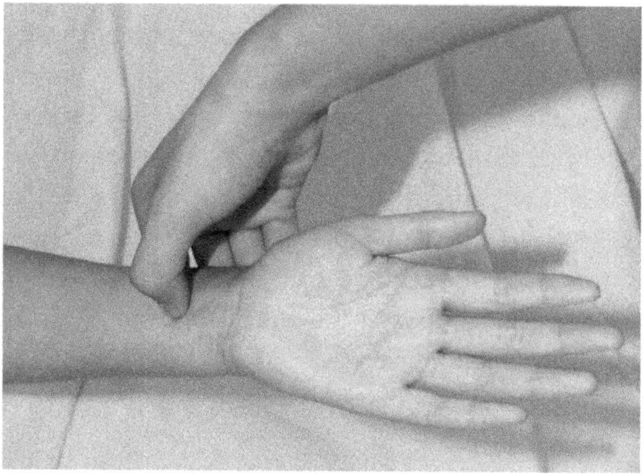

Fig. 2-30

❷ Pressing Hegu

Location

Hegu is located on the back of the hand, between the thumb and first finger, halfway down the 2nd metacarpal, at the bulge of the muscle (Fig. 2-31).

Position

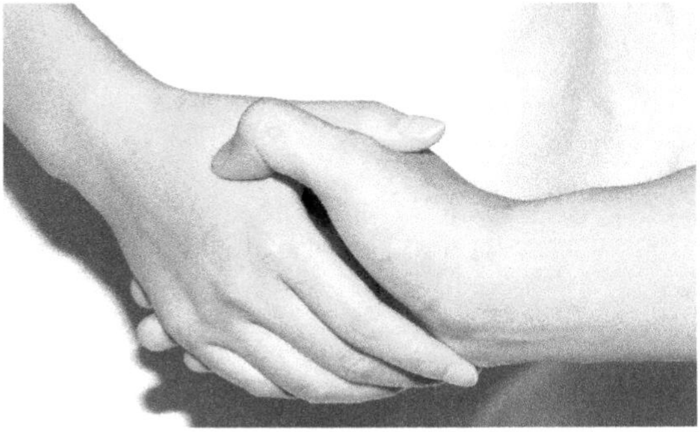

Fig. 2-31

Let your partner sit on the chair or bed.

Technique

Use some force to press Hegu with your thumb for one to five minutes. It can effectively relieve dizziness and nausea.

❸ Pressing Zusanli

Location

Zusanli is located at about 6.5 cm below the depression on the outer side of the knee, about one finger-width lateral to the crest of the

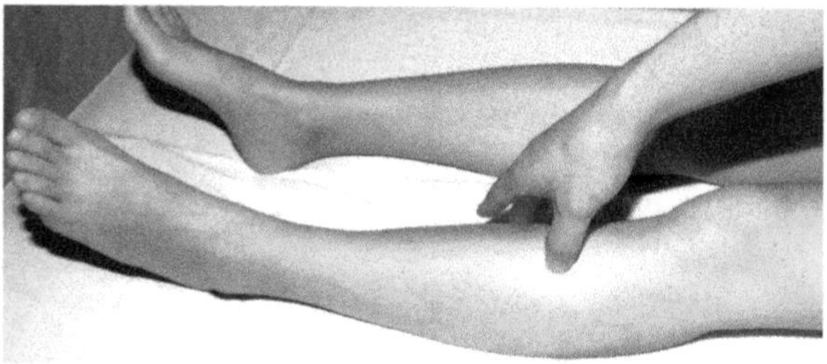

Fig. 2-32

tibia (Fig. 2-32).

Position

Let your partner sit on the chair or bed with his/her knee flexed.

Technique

Press Zusanli for 1 to 5 minutes with your thumb.

Tips

1. Just use as much strength as to induce some soreness and distention.

2. The location may not be too accurate, approximately finding the points should be enough to get results.

3. You can apply the massage when your partner is already affected by carsickness.

Insomnia

Insomnia includes difficulty in going to sleep, shallow sleep, short sleep, waking up too early, insufficient sleep, or sleeping quality being influenced by factors including environment, individual factors body, spirit and mood. According to traditional Chinese medicine, visceral disorders or inner factors can cause insomnia, including weak health, anxiety, depression, and diet. Massage can quiet the spirit, help the communication of heart and kidneys, calm the liver and subdue yang so as to improve insomnia.

Instructions

❶ Pressing Yintang and Taiyang

Location

Yintang is located in between two eyebrows (Fig. 2-33); Taiyang

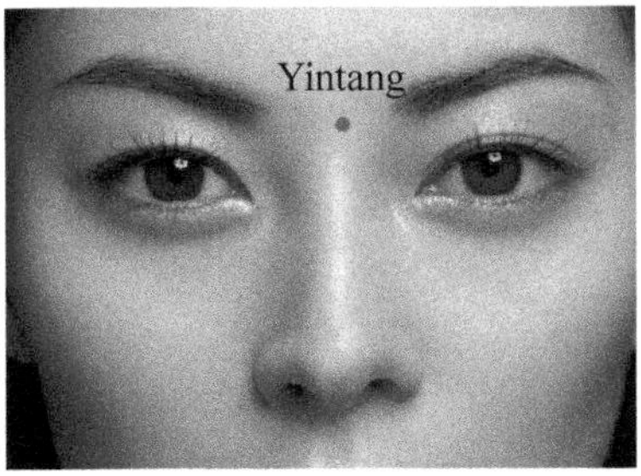

Fig. 2-33

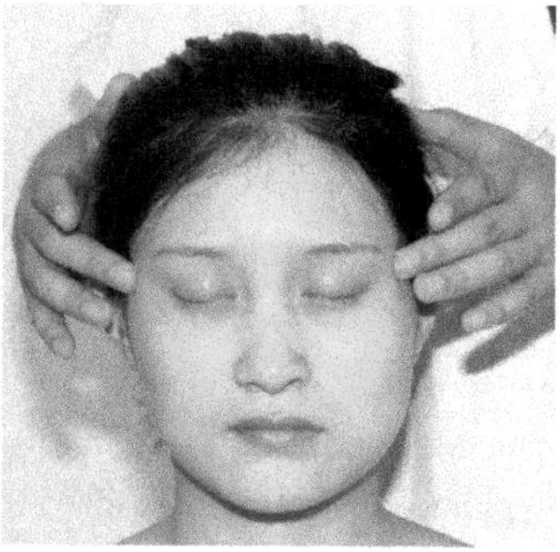

Fig. 2-34

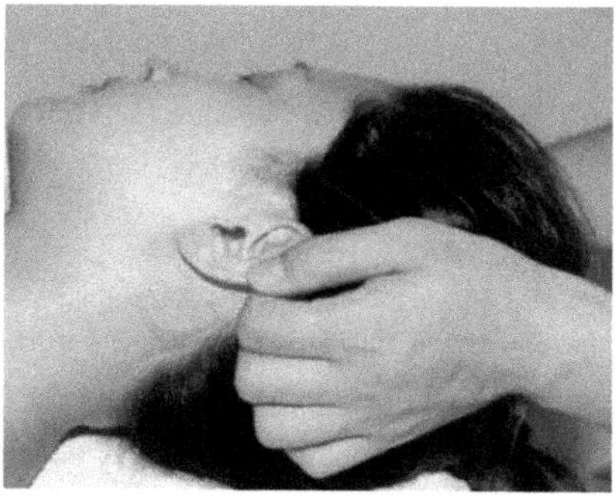

Fig. 2-35

is located in a depression about one finger-width posterior to the lateral end of the eyebrow and the outer canthus (Fig. 2-34).

Position

Let your partner sit on the chair or bed.

Technique

Use your middle fingers to press Yintang 30 times in an upward direction, then press along the bone under the eyebrow and on Taiyang 30 times each.

❷ Manipulations on the ear

Massage the auricle with your index finger from top to bottom, repeat 30 times, then knead the earlobes until they turn reddish (Fig. 2-35).

❸ Manipulations on Anmian point

Location

It is located in the middle of the line connecting the points Yifeng and Fengchi (Fig. 2-36).

Position

Let your partner sit on the chair or bed.

Technique

Massage Anmian 30 times and grasp the neck 30 times until there is a feeling of tension in the nape.

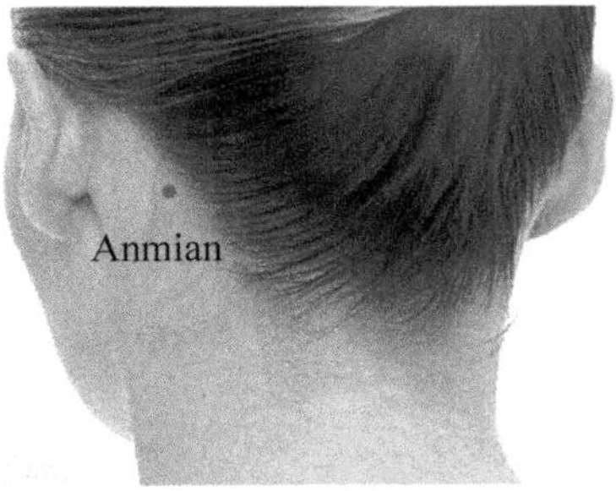

Fig. 2-36

❹ Massage on Yongquan

Location

Yongquan is located on the bottom of the foot, in a depression in between the first third and the back two thirds of the sole of the foot (Fig. 2-37).

Position

Let your partner sit on the chair or bed.

Technique

Use your thumb to press and knead Yongquan 90 times.

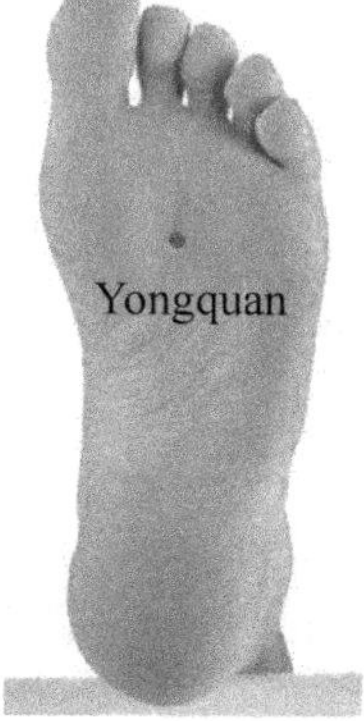

Fig. 2-37

❺ Knead and press Zusanli and Sanyinjiao; Pinch and press Neiguan and Shenmen

Location

Zusanli is located at about 6.5 cm below the depression on the outer side of the knee, about one finger-width lateral to the crest of the tibia (Fig. 2-38). Sanyinjiao is located on the medial side of the

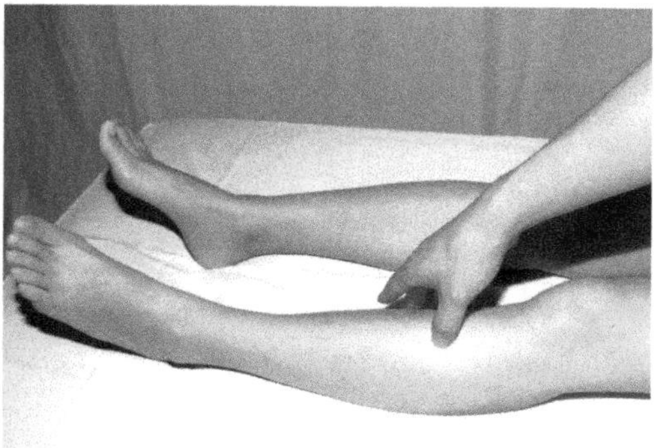

Fig. 2-38

calf, a hand-width above the tip of the inner ankle bone (Fig. 2-39). Neiguan is located at about 6.5 cm above the transverse striation of the wrist, in between the two sinews. Shenmen is located in the depression at the medial side of the transverse striation of the wrist (Fig. 2-40). Jingming is located in a depression slightly above the inner canthus (Fig. 2-41).

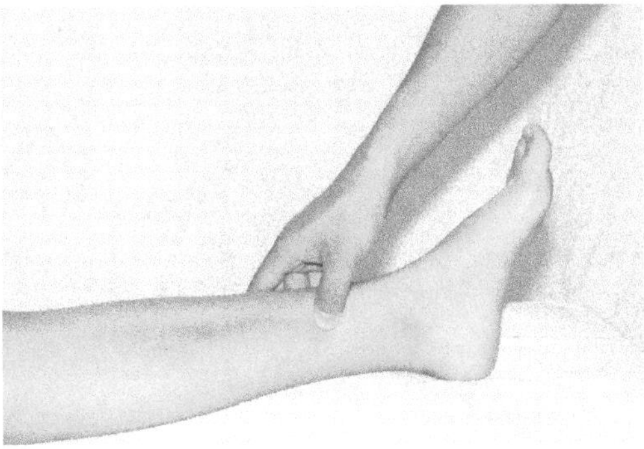

Fig. 2-39

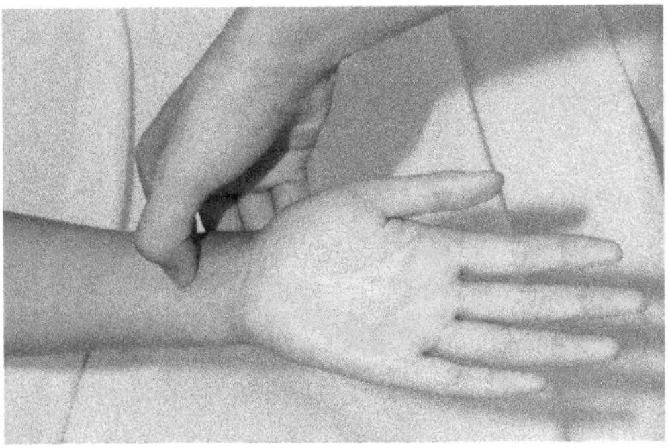

Fig. 2-40

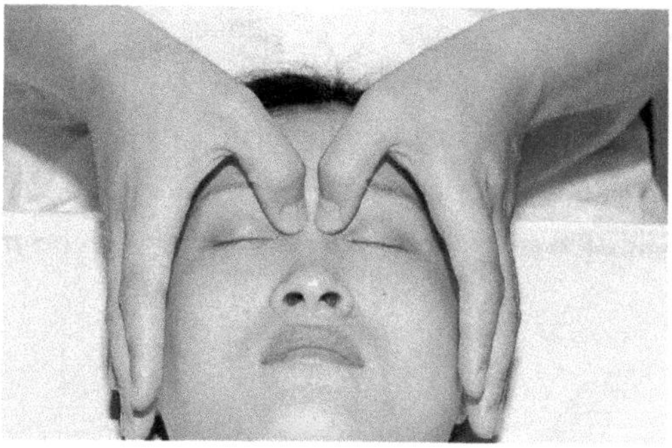

Fig. 2-41

Position

Let your partner sit on the chair or bed.

Technique

Knead Zusanli and Sanyinjiao respectively for one minute every night before going to sleep. Then pinch and press Neiguan and Shenmen for one minute. Knead and rub your partner's back with the palm roots of both hands until there is heat on the skin. To finish off, ask your partner to lie down and calm his/her mind by pressing and kneading Jingming with thumbs and index fingers on both sides for 3 to 5 minutes.

Tips

In order to treat insomnia, tapping, lifting and flicking techniques should not be applied since they easily get people excited. Choose gentle manipulations to calm and quiet your partner's spirit.

Hiccup

Hiccup is usually caused by catching cold after eating or eating too fast.

According to traditional Chinese medicine, hiccup is caused by accumulation of pathogenic qi, sudden rage, improper administration of drugs, eating raw food or eating too fast, which further induce the stomach failing to downbear, so the qi of the stomach and diaphragm moves upward.

It is worth mentioning that patients in critical conditions with obstinate hiccups often present with a bad prognosis, so they should seek treatment as soon as possible.

Massage can resolve spasm and downbear the counter-flowing qi to treat casual occurrence of hiccup.

Instructions

❶ Press Cuanzhu

Location

Cuanzhu is located at the medial boder of the eyebrow (Fig. 2-42).

Position

Let your partner sit on the chair or bed.

Technique

Press Cuanzhu with the pads of both thumbs for about one minute.

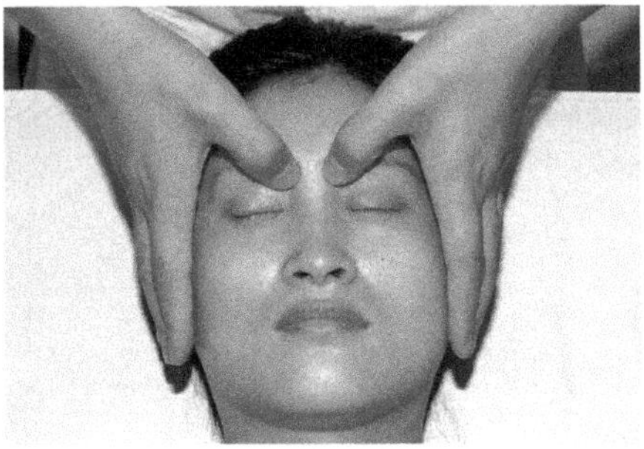

Fig. 2-42

❷ Press and knead Quepen

Location

Quepen is located at the middle of the supraclavicular fossa, about 13 cm off the median line (Fig. 2-43).

Position

Let partner sit on the chair or bed.

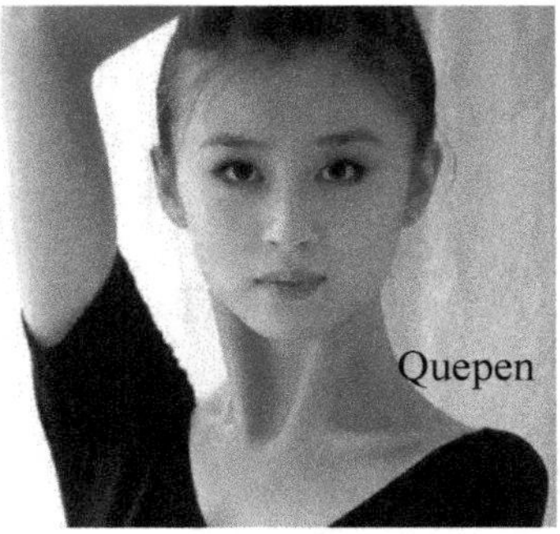

Fig. 2-43

Technique

Press and knead Quepen with the tip of your index finger for around 1 minute until you provoke a feeling of soreness or distention.

❸ Press and knead Danzhong, Zusanli and Neiguan

Location

Danzhong is located on the ventral median line, at the height of the nipples (Fig. 2-44); Zusanli is located at about 6.5 cm below the depression on the outer side of the knee, about one finger-width lateral to the crest of the tibia (Fig. 2-45); Neiguan is located at about 6.5 cm above the transverse striation of the wrist, in between the two sinews (Fig. 2-46).

Position

Let your partner sit on the chair or bed.

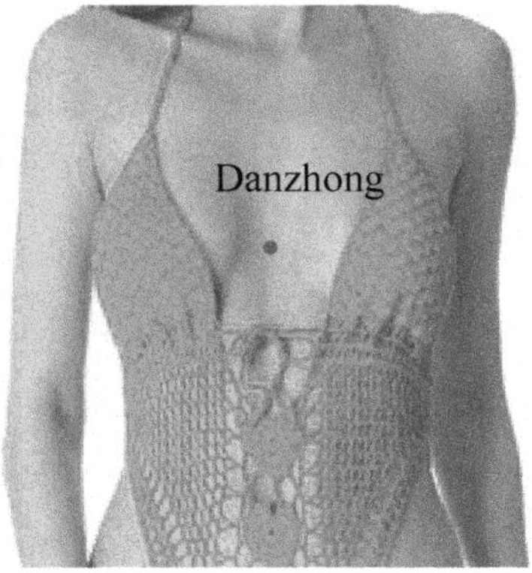

Fig. 2-44

Technique

Press and knead Danzhong, Zusanli and Neiguan respectively for one minute.

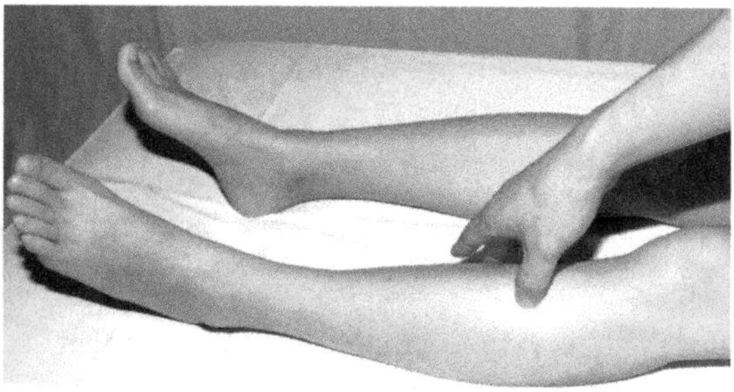

Fig. 2-45

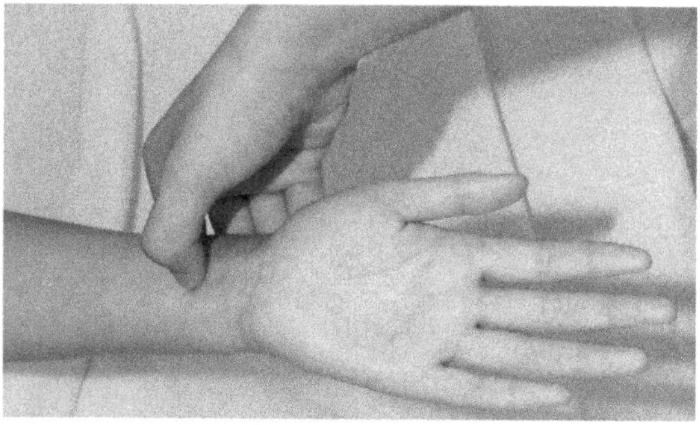

Fig. 2-46

Tips

Use as much strength as possible without causing pain.

Nausea and Vomiting

Vomiting is the reflex taking place when stomach contents reenter the esophagus and are thrown up through the mouth. It can be divided into three phases, namely nausea, dry vomiting and vomiting. Sometimes, there is no sign of nausea or dry vomiting before vomiting. Vomiting is a defensive and protective reflex of the body, it clears harmful substances from the stomach. Although, frequent and intensive vomiting may cause complications of dehydration and electrolyte disturbance.

According to traditional Chinese medicine, nausea and vomiting are caused by an impairment of the downbearing action of the stomach and ascending counterflow of stomach qi.

As for general nausea and vomiting, massage can normalize qi, harmonize the liver and gallbladder, downbear counterflow and check vomiting.

Instructions

❶ Finger-press Juque

Location

Juque is located on the anterior median line, about 20 centimeters above the umbilicus (Fig. 2-47).

Position

Let your partner lie on the bed.

Technique

Kneel down, fold your hands with the fingertips pointing at your partner's neck, press Juque with your middle fingers again and again.

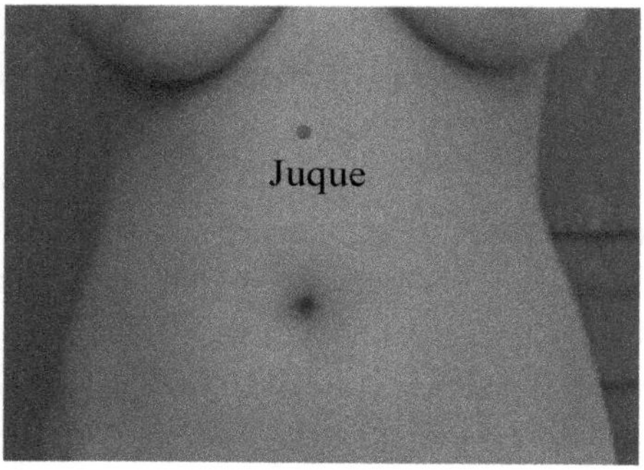

Fig. 2-47

❷ Knead and press Lidui

Location

Lidui is located at the lateral side of the second toe, next to the corner of the nail (Fig. 2-48).

Position

Let your partner sit on the chair or bed.

Technique

Knead and press the Lidui points of both feet.

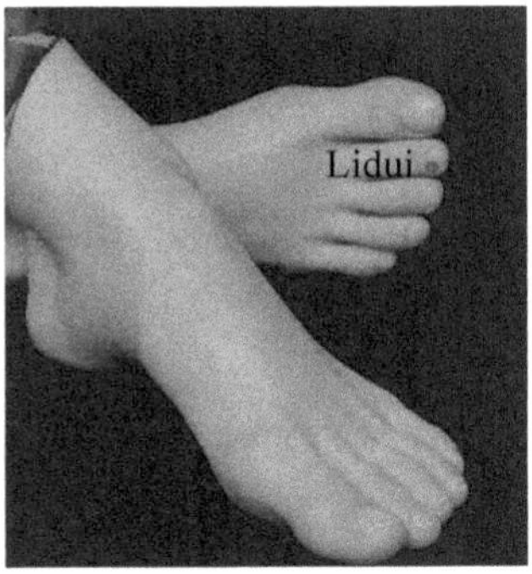

Fig. 2-48

❸ Finger-press Weishu

Location

The location of Weishu is slightly below the middle of the back, 5 centimeters to the side of the twelfth thoracic vertebra (Fig. 2-49).

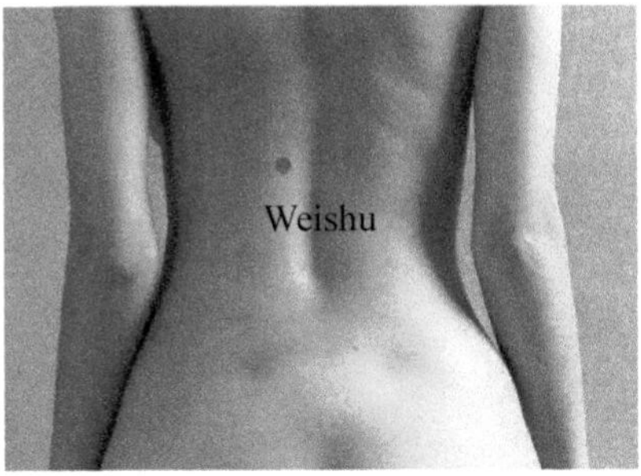

Fig. 2-49

Position

Let your partner lie on his/her stomach.

Technique

Press both hands on your partner's back and use your thumbs to press Weishu on both sides of the spine.

❹ Finger-press Tianshu

Location

Tianshu is located at about 6.5 cm lateral to the umbilicus (Fig. 2-50).

Position

Let your partner lie on the bed.

Technique

Use index, middle and ring ringers of both hands to press the points until there is a slight dent in the fatty tissue.

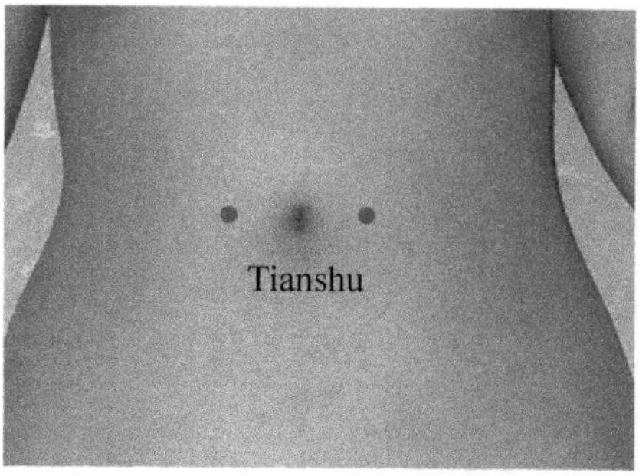

Fig. 2-50

❺ Finger-press Zusanli

Location

Zusanli is located at about 6.5 cm below the depression on the outer side of the knee, about one finger-width lateral to the crest of the tibia (Fig. 2-51).

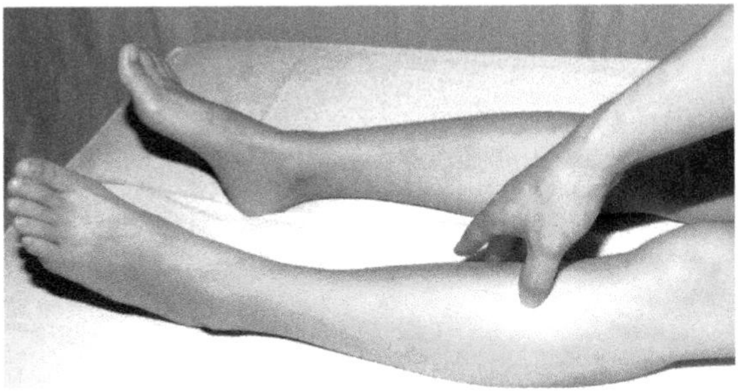

Fig. 2-51

Position

Let your partner lie on the bed.

Technique

Apply finger-pressing on Zusanli on both sides.

❻ Finger-press Baihui

Location

Baihui is the crossover point of the line linking the two ears and the line going through the midpoint of the two eyebrows, namely the top of the head (Fig. 2-52).

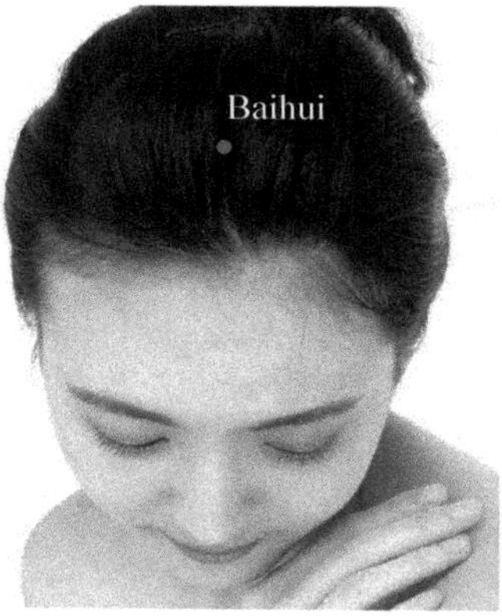

Fig. 2-52

Position

Let your partner sit on the chair or bed.

Technique

Slightly and slowly press Baihui with both thumbs while your hands are holding your partner's head.

Tips

When applying massage, use as much strength as to provoke a sore and distended feeling.

Constipation

Constipation can not really be called a disease, but it can lead to severe damage of the body and cause many diseases, such as hemorrhoids, anal fissure, colon cancer, and even angina, myocardial infarction and cerebral hemorrhage. It can also cause dark skin, acne, intestinal disorders, and pyloric obstruction.

According to traditional Chinese medicine, the essence of food is absorbed when it gets transformed by the spleen and stomach. The waste of this process - the stool - is excreted through the large intestine. When the transportive function of the large intestine is impaired, the stools will stay in the intestines for too long and become dry or hard, leading to constipation. This usually is due to bad life habits, regular massage and a change in diet can help to relieve constipation.

Instructions

❶ Press and knead Tianshu

Location

Tianshu is located at about 6.5 cm to the sides of the umbilicus (Fig. 2-53).

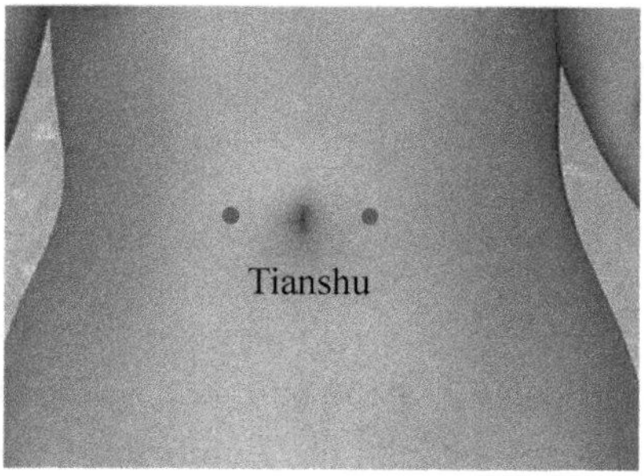

Fig. 2-53

Position

Let your partner lie on the bed.

Technique

Put the pad of your middle finger on Tianshu, press and knead in a clockwise direction for one minute.

❷ Palm knead Zhongwan

Location

Zhongwan is located on the anterior midline of the abodomen, 13 centimeters above the umbilicus (Fig. 2-54).

Position

Let your partner lie on the bed.

Technique

Put your left palm onto Zhongwan, fold your right palm onto the left one to exert strength and conduct kneading and pressing for one minute.

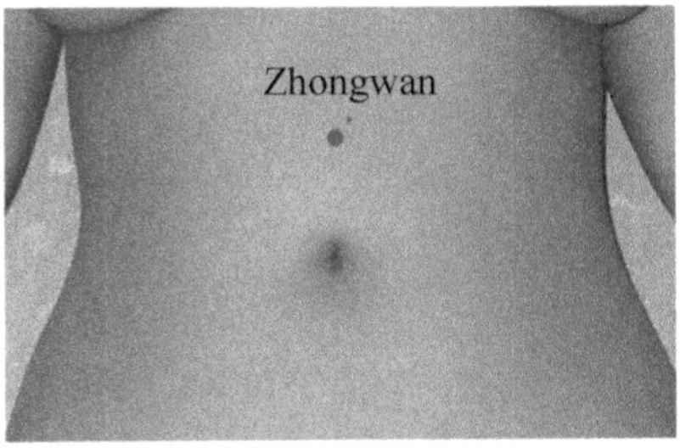

Fig. 2-54

❸ Press and knead Guanyuan

Location

The acupoint is located on the anterior midline , 10 centimeters below the umbilicus (Fig. 2-55).

Position

Let your partner lie on the bed.

Technique

Put the pad of your middle finger on the Guanyuan point, and then press and knead for one minute with appropriate strength.

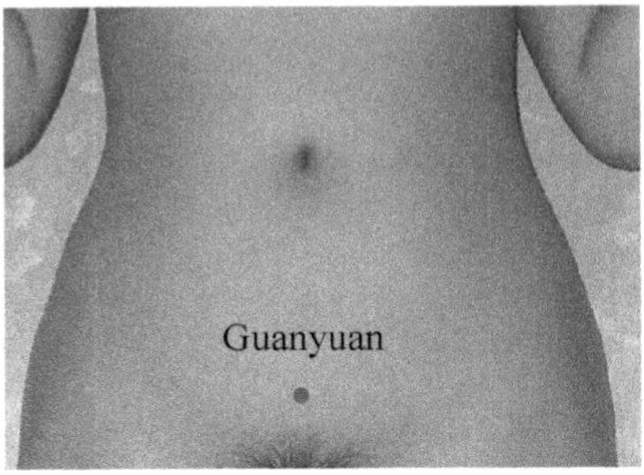

Fig. 2-55

❹ Press and knead Shenshu

Location

Shenshu is located at both sides of the second spinous process of the lumbar vertebrae (Fig. 2-56).

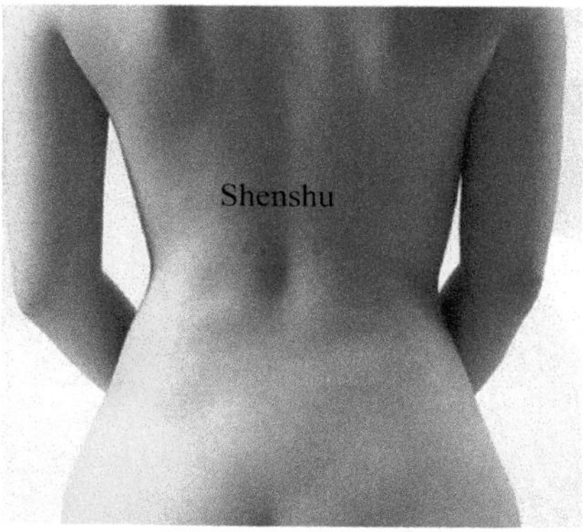

Fig. 2-56

Position

Let your partner lie on the bed or chair, with both hands on the hip.

Technique

Put two thumbs on the Shenshu points of both sides, and then press and knead for one minute with appropriate strength.

❺ Press and knead Hegu

Location

Hegu is located on the back of the hand, between thumb and first finger, halfway down the second metacarpal, at the bulge of the muscle (Fig. 2-57).

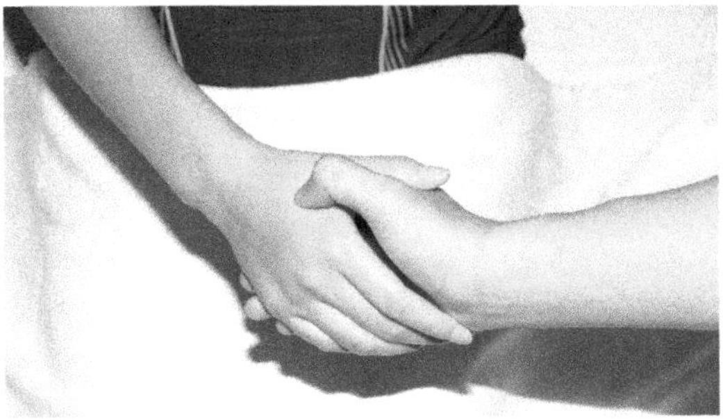

Fig. 2-57

Position

Let your partner sit on the bed or chair.

Technique

Press the Hegu point with the pad of your thumb and knead gently for one minute on each side.

❻ Press and knead Zusanli

Location

Zusanli is located at about 6.5 cm below the depression on the outer side of the knee, about one finger-width lateral to the crest of the tibia (Fig. 2-58).

Position

Let your partner sit on the bed or chair with the knee joints stretched naturally.

Technique

Use your thumbs to press and knead Zusanli for one minute or until your partner feels soreness or distention.

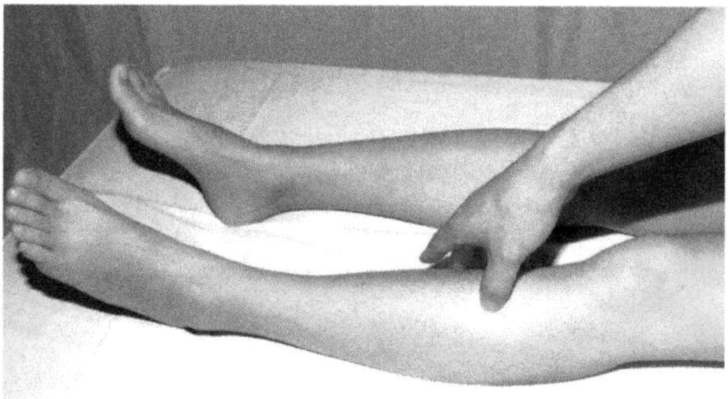

Fig. 2-58

❼ Press and knead Sanyinjiao

Location

Sanyinjiao is located on the medial side of the calf, a hand-width above the tip of the inner ankle bone (Fig. 2-59).

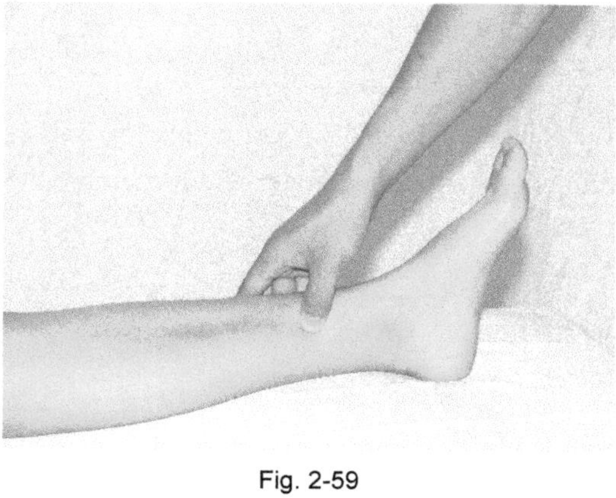

Fig. 2-59

Position

Let your partner sit on the bed or chair with the knee joints stretched naturally.

Technique

Use your thumbs to press and knead Sanyinjiao for one minute with appropriate strength.

Tips

1. Before massage, make sure there are no underlying diseases causing the constipation, such as intestinal obstruction, intestinal adhesion or tumors. Otherwise, you should get treated by a professional doctor.

2. The above massage can regulate the intestinal functions, strengthen abdominal muscles, and improve the constitution. The massage can be applied twice a day, in the morning and evening, and the manipulations should be gentle, flexible, and with a special focus on the abdomen.

Chronic Diarrhea

Diarrhea is a common clinical symptom which refers to an increase of defecation, loose or liquid stools. Consistent diarrhea over two months is called chronic diarrhea, it is usually induced by intestinal inflammation, tumor, improper drug use, mood changes and other diseases that might cause absorption disorders. It is often recurrent and hard to cure, accompanied by abdominal distention, bellyache, and anorexia. Slight diarrhea might happen several times a day, and severe ones might occur over 10 times accompanied by mucus or pus-blood.

According to traditional Chinese medicine, chronic diarrhea is due to factors like invasion of pathogenic qi, mood, uncontrolled diet and innate insufficiency, and that is why people who have great work pressure, an uncontrolled life style, irregular diet and weak constitution will easily get chronic diarrhea.

Massage can clear the heat, resolve accumulation, harmonize the stomach and calm counterflow qi, so as to control diarrhea.

Instructions

❶ Massage Zhongwan and Tianshu

Location

Zhongwan is located on the anterior midline of the abodomen,

13 centimeters above the umbilicus (Fig. 2-60). Tianshu is located at about 6.5 cm to the sides of the umbilicus (Fig. 2-61).

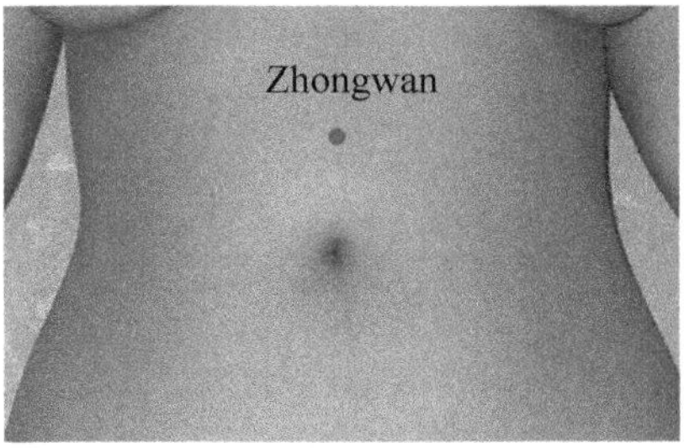

Fig. 2-60

Position

Let your partner lie on the bed.

Technique

Put one hand on top of the other onto your partner's lower abdomen and then upper abdomen, press and knead in an anti-clockwise direction for 3 to 5 minutes. Then finger-knead Zhongwan and Tianshu for one minute each.

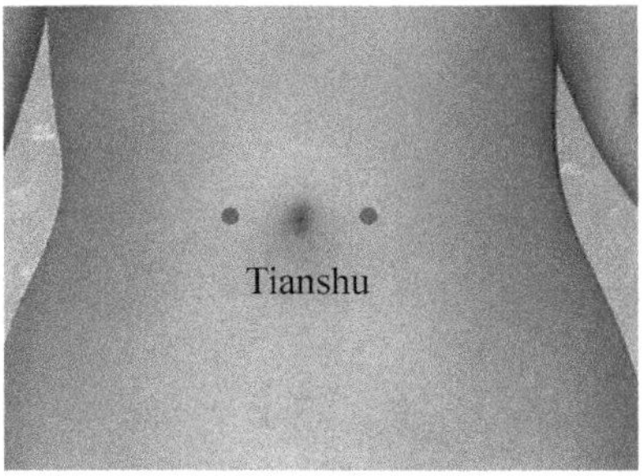

Fig. 2-61

❷ Finger-knead Zusanli

Location

Zusanli is located at about 6.5 cm below the depression on the outer side of the knee, about one finger-width lateral to the crest of the tibia (Fig. 2-62).

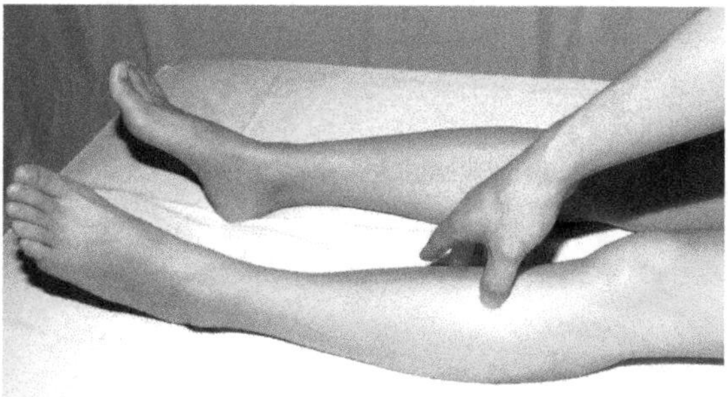

Fig. 2-62

Position

Let your partner sit on the bed or chair.

Technique

Apply finger kneading on Zusanli on both sides for about one minute.

Tips

1. Infectious diarrhea or long time diarrhea with dissatisfactory therapeutic effect should be treated in hospitals.
2. Only massage in a clockwise direction.
3. Try to generate some heat during the massage, let the

belly feel warm.

4. This method can increase the bowel movement and abdominal muscle motion, so it is not suitable to conduct when your partner is starved or stuffed.

5. There might be no obvious effects in the beginning, but continuing use of this method can bring about effects. One massage a day for 30 days can normalize bowel movements.

Abdominal Distention

Abdominal distention is a common symptom of the digestive system, usually occurring in gastrointestinal diseases such as indigestion.

According to traditional Chinese medicine, abdominal distention is caused by spleen-stomach deficiency or stagnation of liver-stomach qi which are induced by abnormal upbearing and downbearing of dynamic qi as well as upbearing counter-flow of turbid qi.

Massage can regulate upbearing and downbearing of dynamic qi, descend counterflow of turbid qi, and promote bowel movements.

Instructions

❶ Press Zhongwan

Location

Zhongwan is located on the anterior midline of the abodomen, 13 centimeters above the umbilicus (Fig. 2-63).

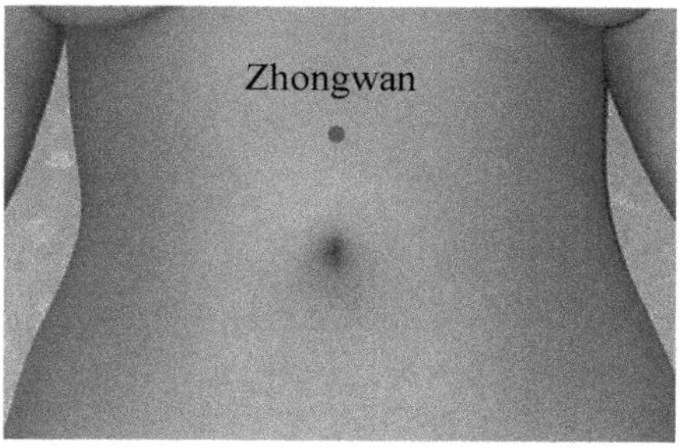

Fig. 2-63

Position

Let your partner sit on the bed or chair.

Technique

Press Zhongwan with the pads of your middle finger and ring finger for 10 times.

❷ Knead and press Tianshu

Location

Tianshu is located at about 6.5 cm to the sides of the umbilicus

(Fig. 2-64).

Position

Let your partner sit on the bed or chair.

Technique

Press Tianshu with the pads of your middle and ring fingers, press in circles and knead the points 20 times each, use appropriate strength.

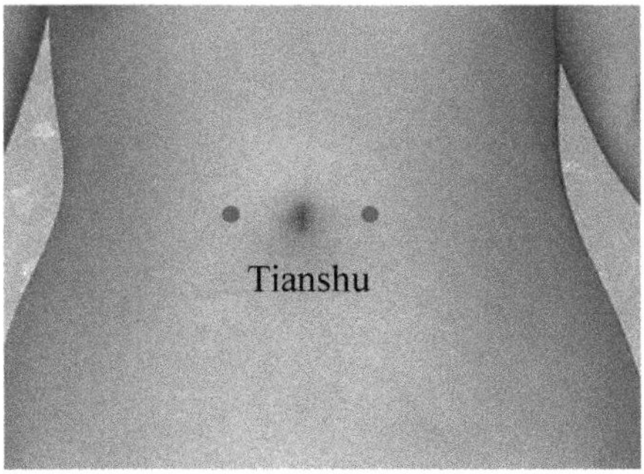

Fig. 2-64

❸ Grasp Hegu

Location

Hegu is located on the back of the hand, between thumb and first finger, halfway down the second metacarpal, at the bulge of the muscle (Fig. 2-65).

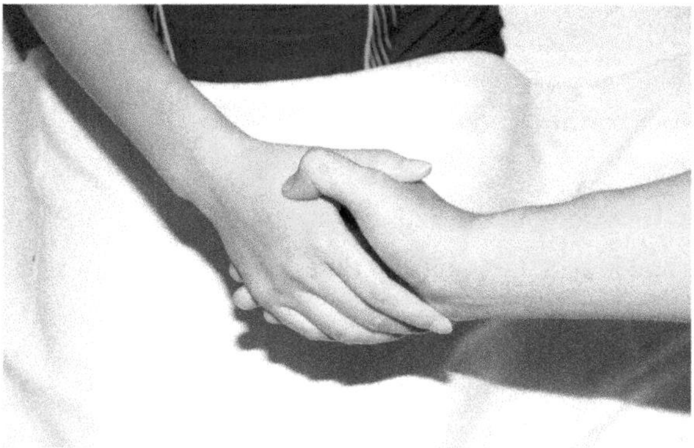

Fig. 2-65

Position

Let your partner sit on the bed or chair.

Technique

Grasp Hegu with thumbs and index fingers, repeat 50 times.

❹ Lift and grasp Jianjing

Location

Jianjing is located on the shoulder, at the midpoint of the line linking Dazhui and the acromion, i.e. the top of shoulder (Fig. 2-66).

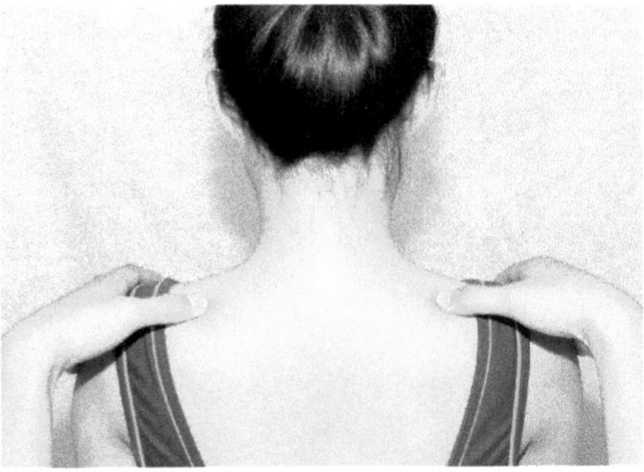

Fig. 2-66

Position

Let your partner sit on the bed or chair.

Technique

Lift and grasp Jianjin with both hands, repeat 50 times.

❺ Pinch and knead Zusanli and Taichong

Location

Zusanli is located at about 6.5 cm below the depression on the outer side of the knee, about one finger-width lateral to the crest of the tibia (Fig. 2-67). Taichong is located on the dorsum of the foot, in a depression distal to the junction of the first and second metatarsal bones (Fig. 2-68).

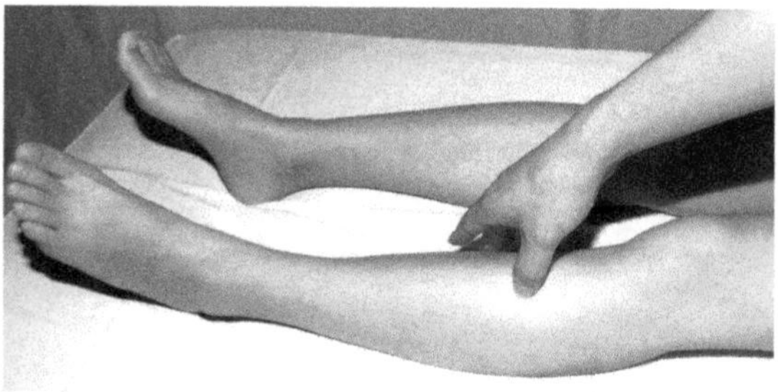

Fig. 2-67

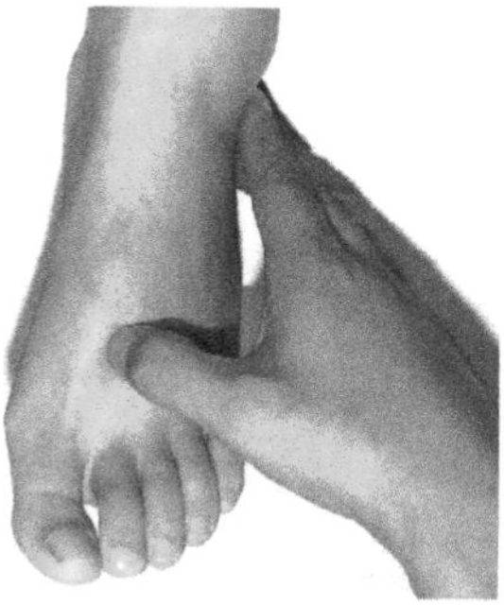

Fig. 2-68

Position

Let your partner sit on the bed or chair.

Technique

Pinch and press Zusanli and Taichong with your thumb.

Tips

The massage is best applied in the evening before sleep with relatively heavy strength.

Hypertension

Hypertension is also called essential hypertension, it is commonly seen among aged people. There are many reasons that can cause hypertension, there are factors such as age, a salty diet, obesity, as well as hereditary, environmental or work-related factors. According to traditional Chinese medicine, hypertension can be caused by long time depression, internal damage and deficiency, overstress, diet, fatigue, a disharmony of liver-kidney yin and yang, induced by over-drinking, age, and life style.

Apart from adjusting emotional moods and taking drugs, massage can be a great preventive measure for hypertension. Massage can regulate the cortex function, improve blood circulation in the brain, dilate the capillaries, strengthen the blood and decrease blood pressure, thus preventing arteriosclerosis and adverse effects of drugs.

Instructions

❶ Massage Yongquan

Location

Yongquan is located on the bottom of the foot, in a depression in between the first third and the back two thirds of the sole of the foot (Fig. 2-69).

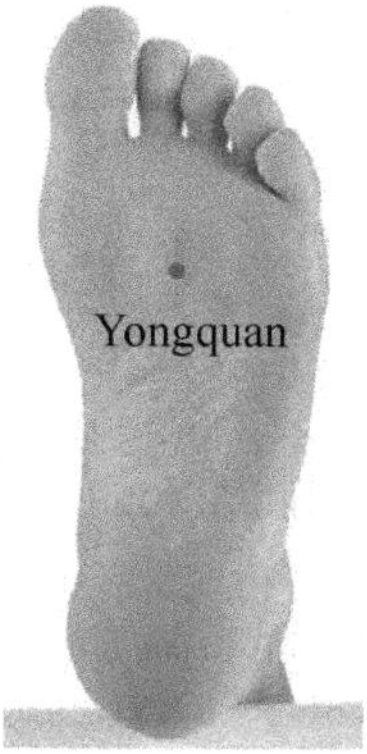

Fig. 2-69

Position

Let your partner sit on the bed or chair.

Technique

Use the thumbs to push from Yongquan to the heel until your partner can feel the heat, repeat 100 times once or twice a day.

The direction of the massage is towards the toes, don't do it the other way round. Clinically, massage on Yongquan is usually combined with a foot bath. For example, one of the most famous four doctors in Beijing, Dr. Shi Jinmo, has a Sichuan pepper foot bath every evening, followed by left hand massage on the right foot and right hand massage on the left foot, 100 times each. Dr. Shi believes that leading the heat downward can strengthen the body.

❷ Press and knead Yinlingquan

Location

Yinlingquan is located at the inside of the knee, in a depression inferior and posterior to the medial condyle of the tibia (Fig. 2-70).

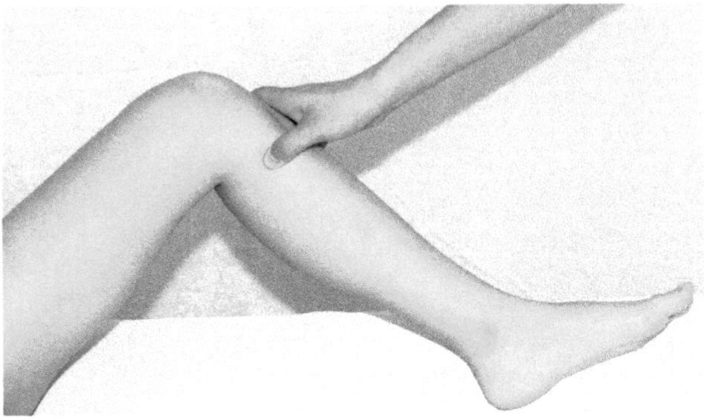

Fig. 2-70

Position

Let your partner sit on the bed or chair.

Technique

Press and knead Yinlingquan in a clockwise direction for around two minutes, and then in the other direction for another two minutes, until your partner feels soreness and distention.

❸ Press and knead Quchi

Location

Quchi is on the end of the lateral side of the transverse elbow

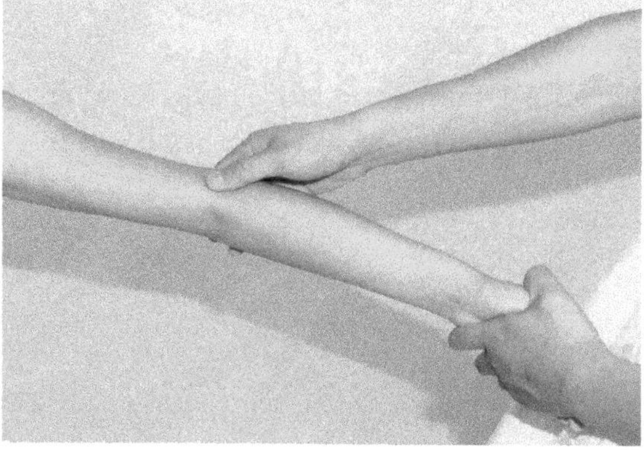

Fig. 2-71

striation when the elbow is flexed (Fig. 2-71).

Position

Let your partner sit on the bed or chair.

Technique

Use your thumb to press and knead Quchi in a clockwise direction for two minutes, and then another two minutes in an anti-clockwise direction. Your partner should feel some local soreness and distention.

❹ Press and knead Sanyinjiao

Location

Sanyinjiao is located at the medial side of the calf, about one hand-width above the tip of the inner ankle bone (Fig. 2-72).

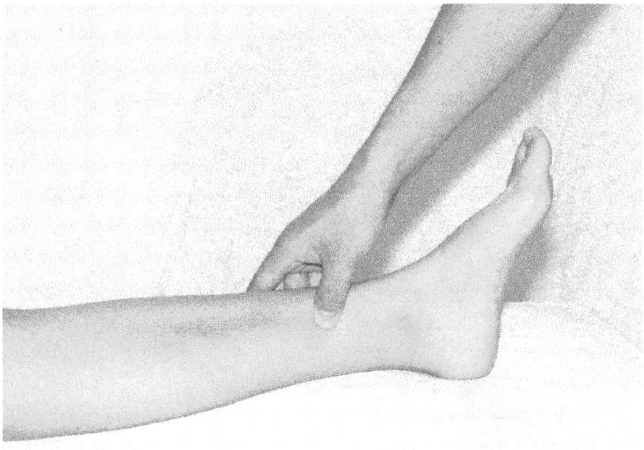

Fig. 2-72

Position

Let your partner sit on the bed or chair.

Technique

Use your thumb to press and knead Sanyinjiao in a clockwise direction for two minutes, and then another two minutes in an anti-clockwise direction. Your partner should feel some local soreness and distention.

❺ Knead and grasp Fengchi

Location

Fengchi is located below the occipital bone on the neck, in a depression between sternocleidomastoid and trapezius (Fig. 2-73).

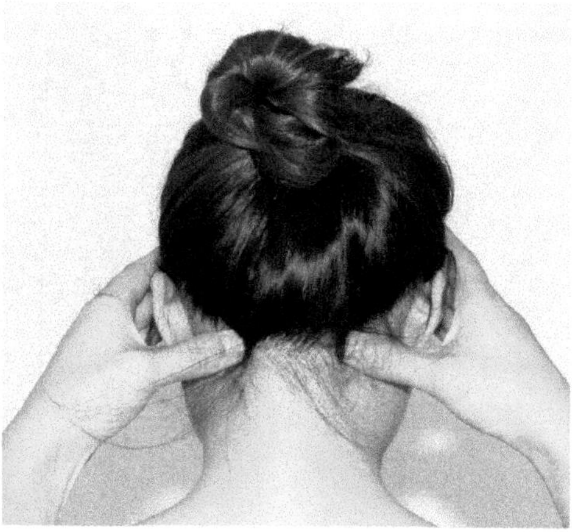

Fig. 2-73

Position

Let your partner lie on his/her stomach.

Technique

Knead and grasp Fengchi with thumb and index finger. Your partner should feel some local soreness and distention.

❻ Press and knead Baihui

Location

Baihui is the crossover point of the line linking the two ears and the line going through the midpoint of the two eyebrows, namely the top of the head (Fig. 2-74).

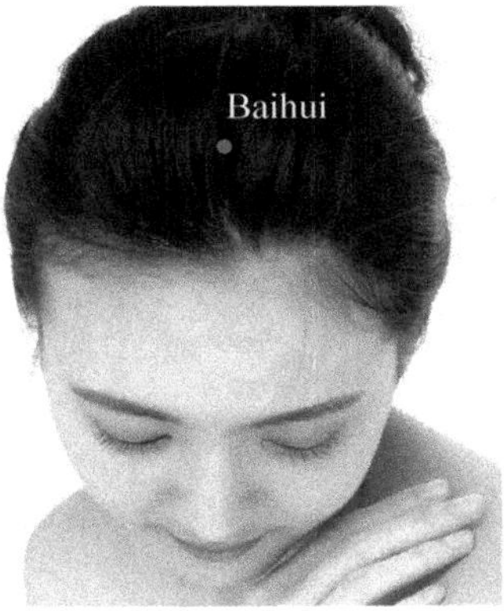

Fig. 2-74

Position

Let your partner lie on the bed.

Technique

Press Baihui with your thumb for half an minute, then press and knead the point for one minute in a clockwise direction, then in the other direction for another minute. Your partner should feel some local soreness and distention.

❼ Press and knead Taichong

Location

Taichong is located on the dorsum of the foot, in a depression distal to the junction of the first and second metatarsal bones (Fig. 2-75).

Position

Let your partner sit on the bed or chair.

Technique

Hold the forefoot, finger-press Taichong with your thumb or index finger, then press and knead the point in a clockwise direction for one minute and then in an anti-clockwise direction for another one minute.

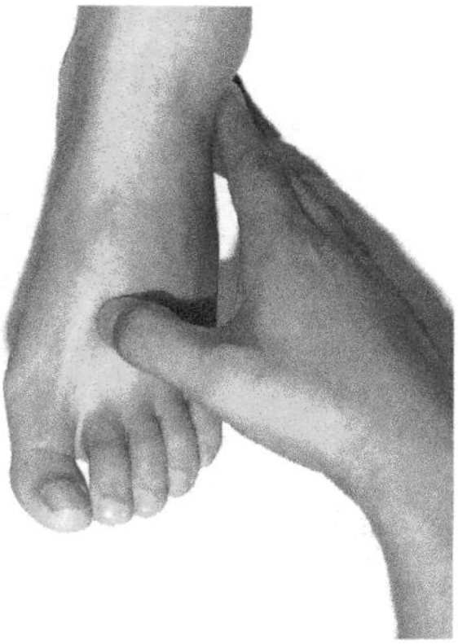

Fig. 2-75

❽ Finger-press Taixi

Location

Taixi is located at the medial side of the foot, right behind the medial malleolus, in the depression between the tip of the medial malleolus and the Achilles tendon (Fig. 2-76).

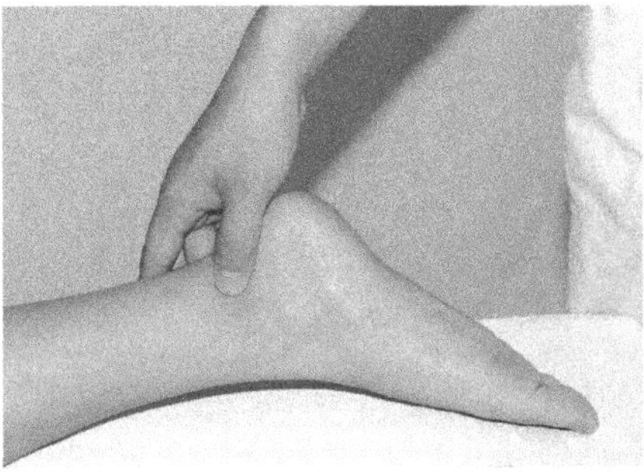

Fig. 2-76

Position

Let your partner sit on the bed or chair.

Technique

Hold your partner's ankle, and press Taiyi with your thumb for one minute, then press and knead the point in a clockwise direction for one minute and then in an anti-clockwise direction for another minute. Your partner should feel some local soreness and distention.

Tips

Regularly doing some of the described manipulations can help to prevent the occurrence of hypertension.

✿ Stiff Neck

Stiff neck is a common disease with soreness and pain of the neck and back, limitation of neck motion, sometimes there are no symptoms before sleeping. It can be caused by an improper posture of the head and neck during sleep or an inappropriate pillow or wind cold invading the neck.

According to traditional Chinese medicine, stiff neck is due to sprain of the neck or invasion of pathogenic wind, cold or dampness which can cause a stagnation of blood and qi, as well as obstruction of meridians.

Massage can resolve the spasm, regulate qi and stop pain.

Instructions

❶ Press and knead tender points (Ashi point)

Location

Ashi points here refer to the tender points in the neck area (mostly located in the sternocleidomastoid muscle, trapezius, etc.) (Fig. 2-77).

Position

Let your partner sit on the bed or chair.

Technique

Put your index, middle and ring finger of your right or left hand

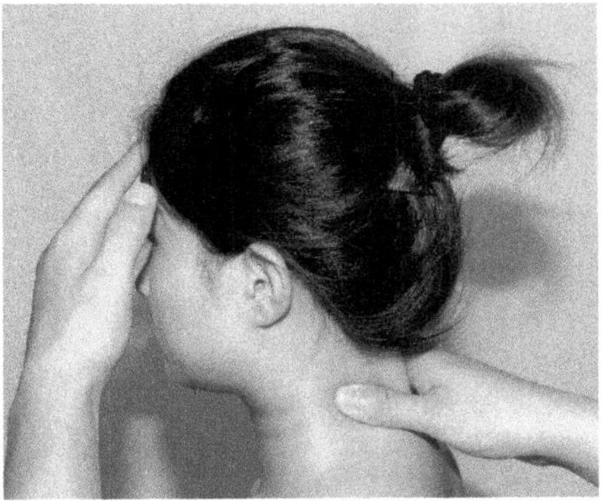

Fig. 2-77

together, press and knead the tenderness for around 5 minutes with gradually increasing strength. Right hand and left hand can alternately conduct the massage.

❷ Grasp Fengchi and Jianjing

Location

Fengchi is located below the occipital bone on the neck, in a depression between sternocleidomastoid and trapezius. Jianjing is

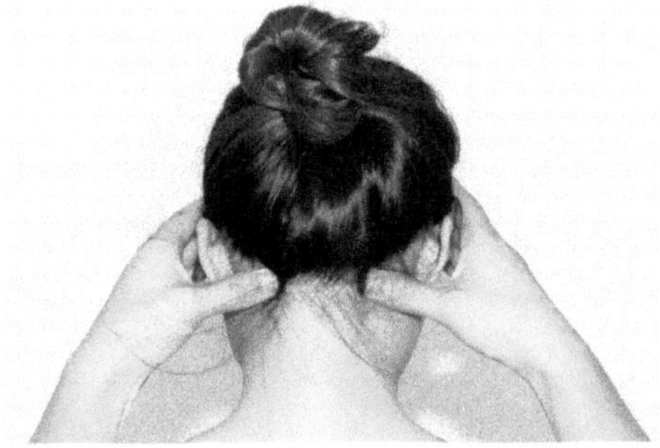

Fig. 2-78

located on the shoulder, on the midpoint of the line linking Dazhui and the acromion, i.e. the top of the shoulder (Fig. 2-79).

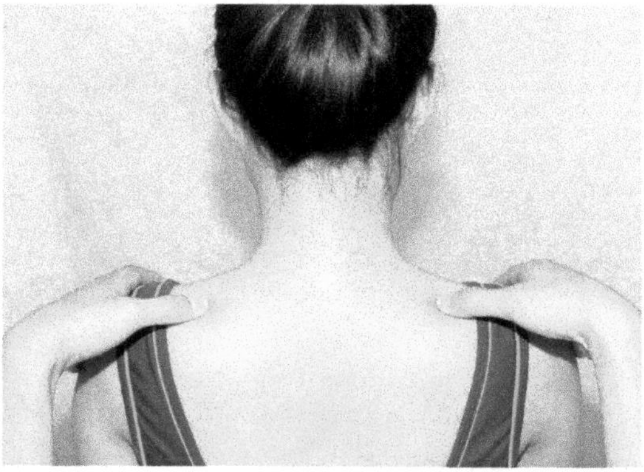

Fig. 2-79

Position

Let your partner sit on the bed or chair.

Technique

Grasp Fengchi and Jianjing on both sides with your thumb and index finger for one to two minutes each.

❸ Finger-press Laozhen (Extrapoint)

Location

Laozhen is located on the dorsum of the hand, between the second and third metacarpal bones, about one centimeter proximal to the metacarpophalangeal joint (Fig. 2-80).

Position

Let your partner sit on the bed or chair.

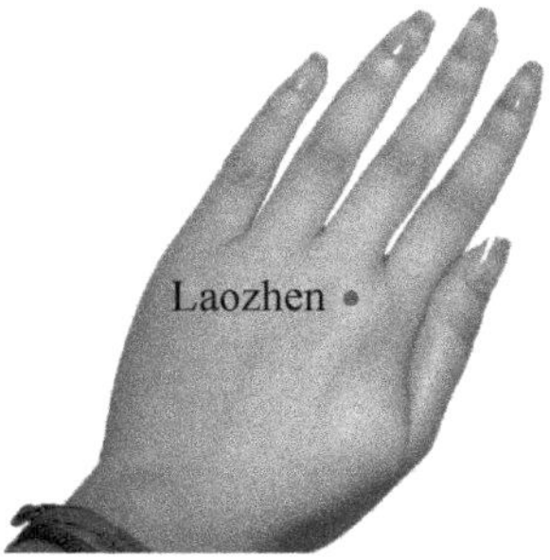

Fig. 2-80

Technique

Use your thumb or index finger to press Liaozhen. When your partner feels soreness or distention, continue for another two to three minutes.

Tips

1. After finishing the above techniques, you can also do some manipulations on the head and neck, like forward and backward flexion, twisting and rotating, watch out to be gentle and slow.

2. Pay attention to the differentiation of stiff neck and early cervical spondylopathy, which requires treatment in hospital.

3. Detailed diagnosis and treatment are required for recurring short term stiff necks. If a stiff neck is accompanied by headache, dizziness, finger numbness, and arm pain, it might be induced by cervical spondylopathy which needs inspection in hospital as early as possible.

✿ Scapulohumeral Periarthritis

Scapulohumeral periarthritis refers to periarthritis of the shoulder, which is caused by chronic inflammation of the shoulder muscles, tendon, bursa synovialis, joint capsule and other soft tissues. It causes internal and external adhesion of the shoulder joint, pain around the shoulder and impairment of movement.

According to Chinese Medicine, this disease results from being affected mainly by pathogenic wind, cold pathogen and dampness. It causes pain around the shoulder and impairs movement; therefore it is called "rheumatism of exposed shoulder".

Massage has very good effects in relieving scapulohumeral periarthritis by relaxing the muscles and tendons, promoting the flow of qi and blood and relieving pain.

Instructions

❶ Massage the upper limb and shoulder

Take this as preparation method. Please let your partner sit upright on the bed or chair. Massage with your right palm from the partner's wrist, via elbow and shoulder to the neck, from inside to outside and backside of the upper limb and shoulder. Repeat 20-30 times (Fig. 2-81).

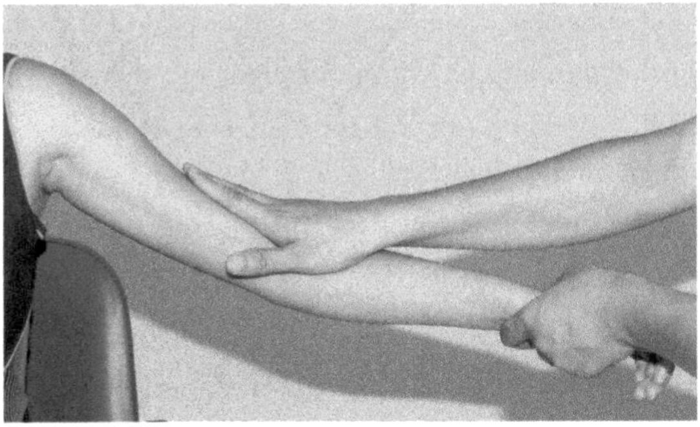

Fig. 2-81

❷ Roll the shoulder and the upper limb

Please let your partner lie on the bed or sit on a chair. Roll or knead the front side of the diseased shoulder and the inner side of the upper limb. Repeat this for several times, and combine with stretching and outward turning of the upper limb. Let your partner lie down,

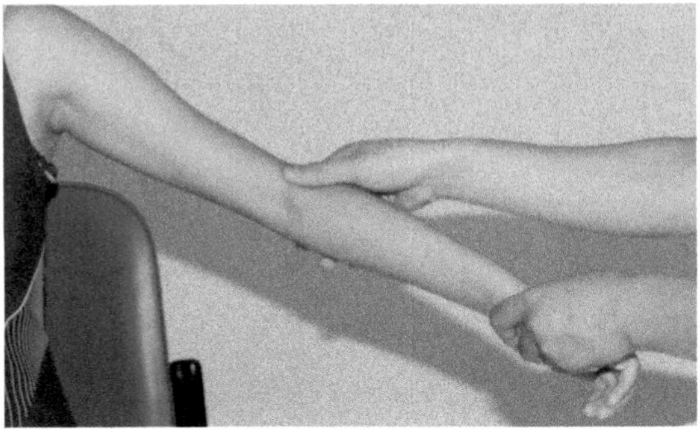

Fig. 2-82

hold his or her elbow with one hand and roll the shoulder with your other hand. Ask your partner to lift and adduct the limb. Then let your partner lie on his/her back, massage the upper part of the chest and the front side of the shoulder by rolling or pressing; then let your partner sit up and stretch the limb towards the back (Fig. 2-82).

❸ Press Hegu, Quchi and Jianjing

Location

Hegu is located on the back of the hand, between thumb and first finger, halfway down the second metacarpal, at the bulge of the muscle (Fig. 2-83). Quchi is on the end of the lateral side of the transverse elbow striation when the elbow is flexed (Fig. 2-84). Jianjing is located on the shoulder, on the midpoint of the line linking Dazhui and the acromion, i.e. the top of the shoulder (Fig. 2-85).

Please let your partner sit on the bed or chair. Press Hegu, Quchi,

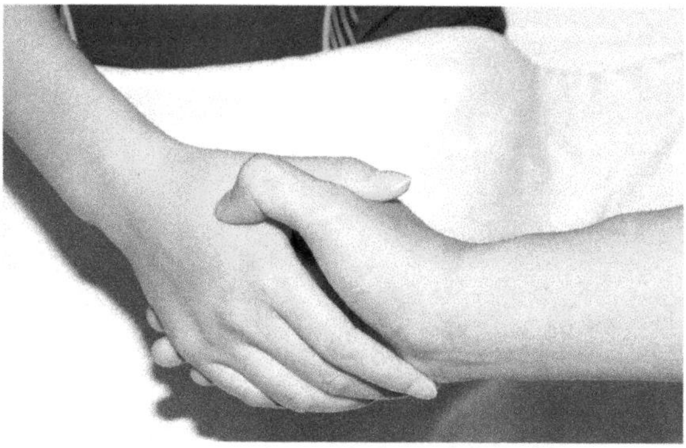

Fig. 2-83

Quepen, Jiandu, Jianzhen, Jianqia, Jianjing,Tianzong, Quyuan and Ashi points in this sequence until your partner can feel some soreness and distention.

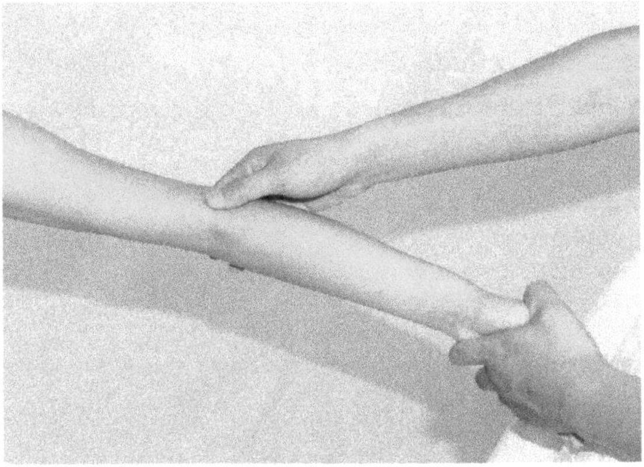

Fig. 2-84

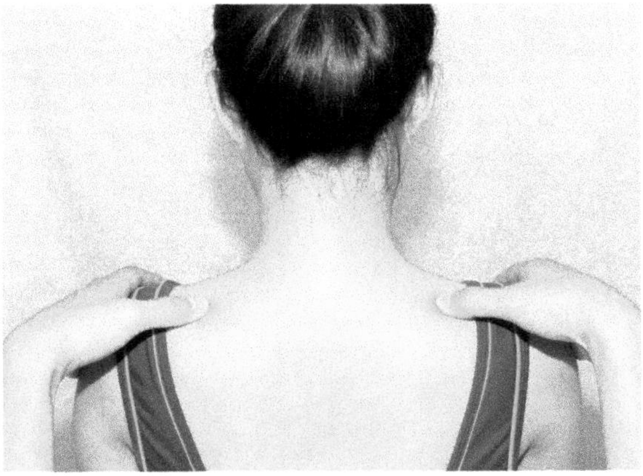

Fig. 2-85

❹ Rotate the shoulder

Please let your partner sit on the bed or chair. Stand behind the affected side of your partner; hold his/her shoulder with one hand and hold the wrist or elbow with the other hand, rotate the affected shoulder around the shoulder joint. Gradually increase the size of the movement. Then hold the forearm with one hand to bend the elbow and adduct the forearm. Rotate the forearm in a circle to the other shoulder, the top of the head and back down, repeat ten times. Meanwhile, hold and pinch the affected shoulder with the other hand (Fig. 2-86).

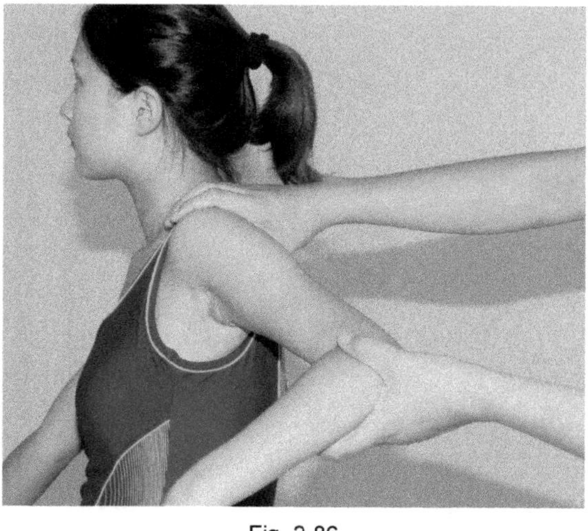

Fig. 2-86

❺ Lift and shake the upper limb

Please let your partner sit on the bed or chair. Stand beside the affected shoulder of your partner and hold the wrist of the affected arm. Let your partner lower the shoulder and bend the elbow; shake it while lifting the arm. Enlarge movement scope gradually and increase your force. Please pay attention not to overexert yourself (Fig. 2-87).

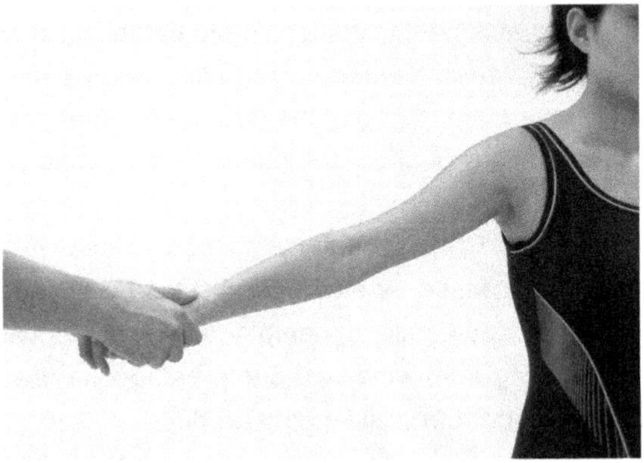

Fig. 2-87

Tips

1. Patients with scapulohumeral periarthritis often have a cold feeling in the shoulder. So before your massage it please use a hot towel to cover the neck and shoulder in order to enhance the effect.

2. Massage the back of the hand from the fingers to the shoulder with forefinger, middle finger, ring finger and little finger; then massage the palm in the opposite direction. A towel can also be used as massage tool. Repeat 3 to 5 times until the skin starts to turn red.

✿ Cervical Spondylosis

Cervical spondylosis is a common disease which is caused by internal and external factors leading to pathological changes of the cervical vertebrae and surrounding nerves and blood vessels. People suffering from this disease will feel pain in the neck and shoulders or show symptoms of headache and limb paralysis.

According to Chinese medicine, most cases of cervical spondylosis are caused by strain of muscles and bones, stagnation of qi and blood, phlegm-damp and blockage of veins and tendons, resulting from wind-cold-damp pathogens obstructing the qi and blood or from constant overwork.

Massage can relax the muscles and stimulate the blood circulation, having a sound treatment effect on cervical spondylosis. The symptoms can be relieved after massage.

Instructions

❶ Press Taiyang from both sides

Location

Taiyang is located at the tempora of the head, in the depression at a finger's width behind the outer tip of the brow and the outer corner of the eye, near the hairline (Fig. 2-88).

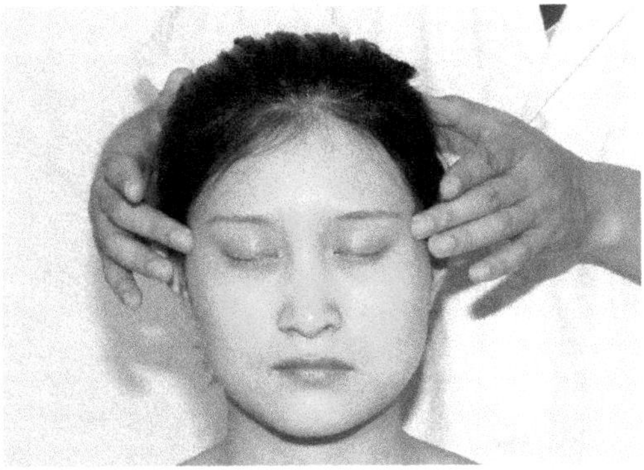

Fig. 2-88

Position

Let your partner sit on the chair.

Technique

Stand in front of your partner, put your thumbs onto both Taiyang points of your partner, separate your fingers on each side of the head, and press the two Taiyang points at the same time, repeat 20-30 times.

❷ Press Baihui

Location

Baihui is the highest point of the head, at the point of intersection of a straight line between the two ears and a straight line coming up from in between the eyebrows (Fig. 2-89).

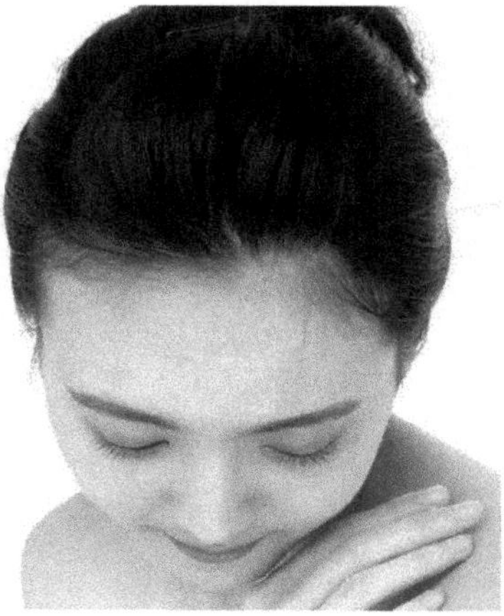

Fig. 2-89

Position

Let your partner sit on the chair.

Technique

Press the Baihui with middle finger or forefinger with increasing strength, repeat 20-30 times.

❸ Press Fengchi

Location

Fengchi is located below the occipital bone on the neck, in a depression between sternocleidomastoid and trapezius (Fig. 2-90).

Position

Let your partner sit on the chair.

Technique

Use both thumbs to press Fengchi on one side only with the other

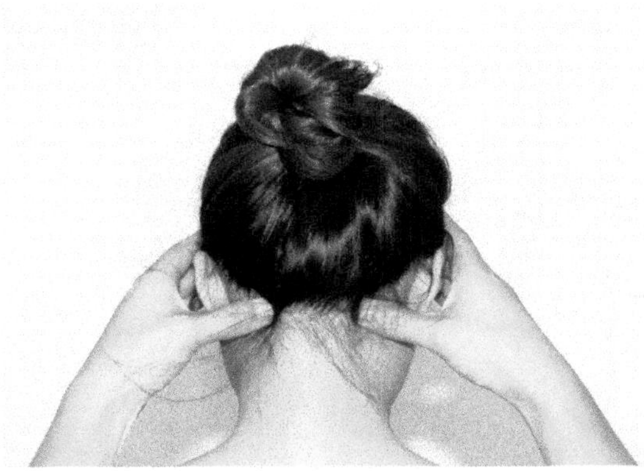

Fig. 2-90

fingers on the sides of the head. Slowly increase the strength, repeat 20-30 times.

❹ Massage cervical muscles and press Fengchi and Dazhui

Location

Fengchi is located below the occipital bone on the neck, in a depression between sternocleidomastoid and trapezius. Dazhui is located at the lower part of the neck, in the depression under the 7th cervical spinous process (Fig. 2-91).

Position

Let your partner sit on the chair.

Technique

Put your hands on your partner's neck with both thumbs on the same side and the other fingers on the opposite side of the cervical muscles. Clench your hands to lift the cervical muscles and pull them backwards, relax your grip and massage from Fengchi downward to Dazhui, repeat 20-30 times (Fig. 2-92).

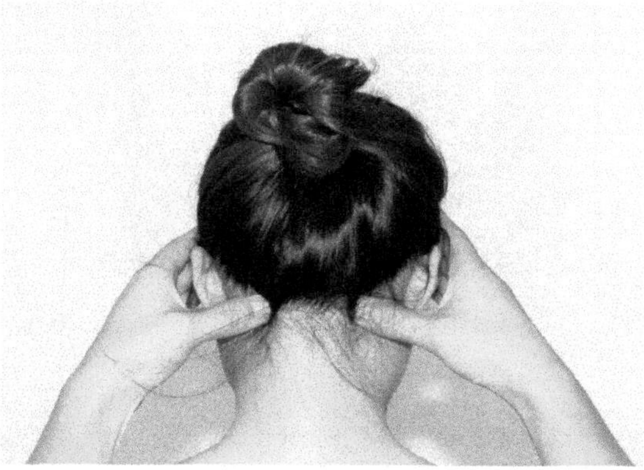

Fig. 2-91

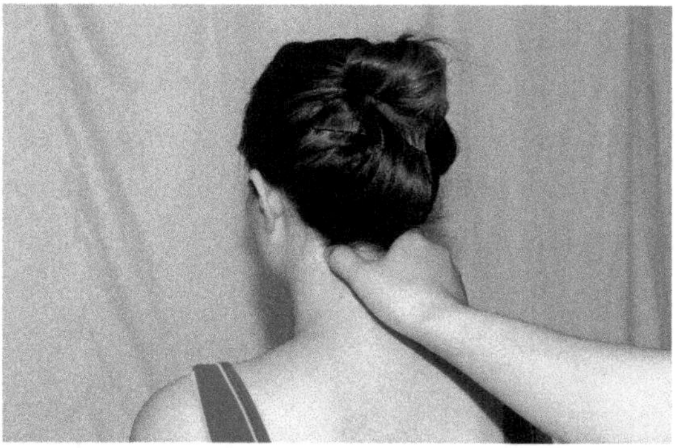

Fig. 2-92

❺ Press Jianjing

Location

Jianjing is located on the shoulder, on the midpoint of the line linking Dazhui and the acromion, i.e. the top of the shoulder (Fig. 2-93).

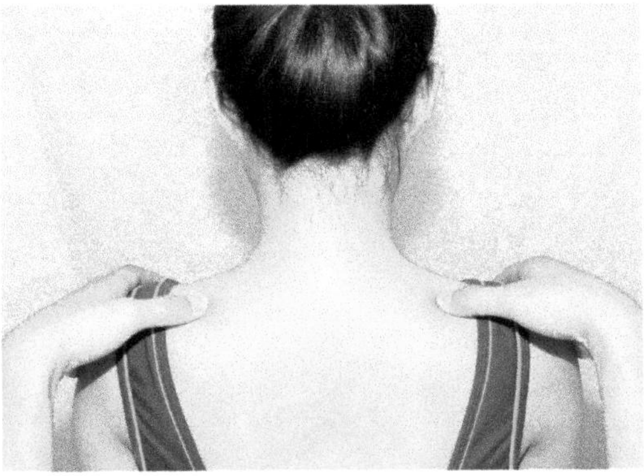

Fig. 2-93

Position

Let your partner sit on the chair.

Technique

Use the pads of your middle fingers to alternately press Jianjing on both sides, increase the pressure, repeat 10-20 times.

❻ Press Dazhui

Location

Dazhui is located at the lower part of the neck, in the depression under the 7th cervical spinous process. If the location of the spinous process is not obvious, please let your partner move his/her neck - the bone which is not moving is the first thoracic vertebra, level with the shoulder (Fig. 2-94).

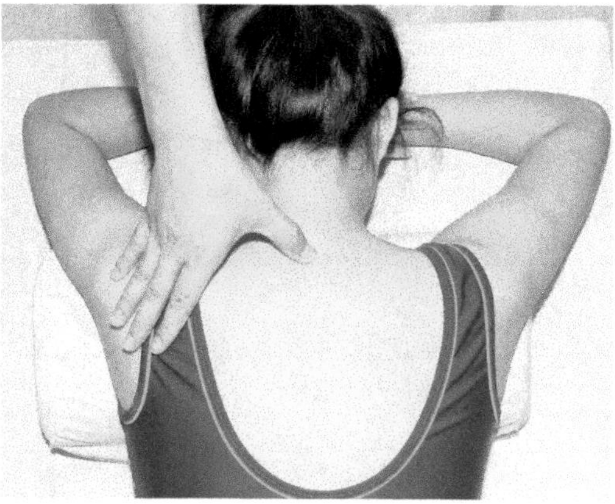

Fig. 2-94

Position

Let your partner sit on the chair.

Technique

Put your hand on your partner's upper back and keep your fingers together. Massage Dazhui until your partner can feel some heat.

❼ Press Neiguan and Waiguan

Location

Let your partner extend his/her arm and turn the palm up, Neiguan is located at about 6.5 cm above the inner wrist crease, in between the two central tendons (Fig. 2-95). Waiguan is on the other side of it, at about 6.5 cm above the outer wrist crease, between the radius and ulna (Fig. 2-96).

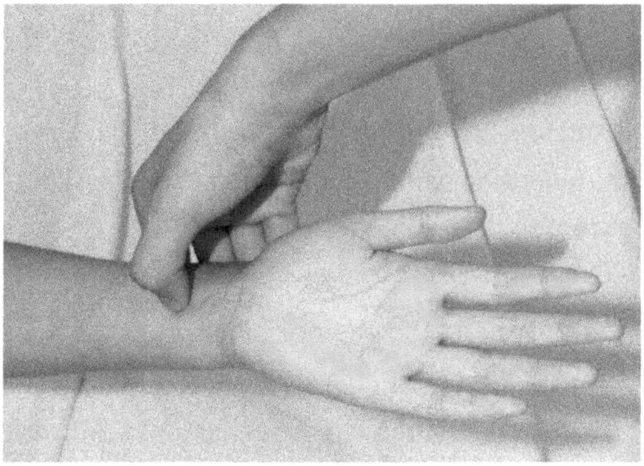

Fig. 2-95

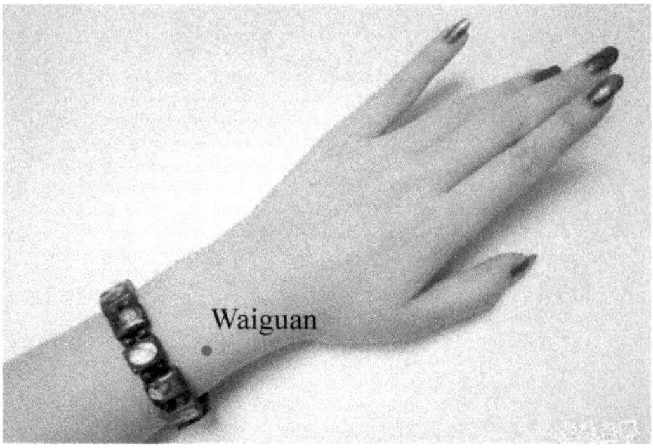

Fig. 2-96

Position

Let your partner sit on the chair.

Technique

Put your thumb tip on Neiguan and middle finger on Waiguan. Press them at the same time for 0.5-1 minute. Then change to the other hand.

❽ Massage Hegu

Location

Hegu is located on the back of the hand, between thumb and first finger, halfway down the second metacarpal, at the bulge of the muscle (Fig. 2-97).

Position

Let your partner sit on the chair or bed.

Technique

Press Hegu with the thumb tip, repeat 10-20 times, then change to the other hand.

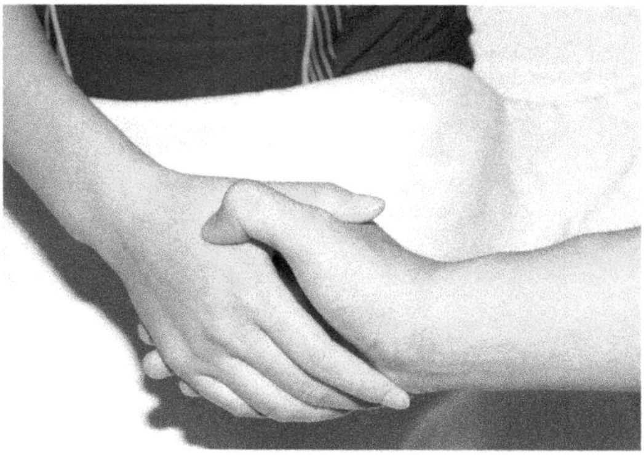

Fig. 2-97

Tips

1. Massage each point for around 20 minutes and make sure that the patient feels comfortable.

2. Massage softly and gently, otherwise your partner will feel uncomfortable.

Lumbago and Backache

Lumbago and backache is not a disease in itself, but a common and shared symptom of many diseases. Any lesion of the skin, subcutaneous tissue, muscles, ligaments, spine, ribs, spinal cord and spinal meninges of the waist and back can cause lumbago and backache.

According to Chinese medicine, lumbago and backache falls into the categories of exogenous diseases or internal injuries. Most exogenous diseases are caused by external pathogenic wind and cold or disharmony of qi and blood. It often presents with sudden and intense pain in the waist and back, which leads to pain when bending over and lying down.

Massage can regulate qi and blood, yin and yang, promote the flow of qi and blood, activate blood circulation and remove blood stasis, relieve swelling and pain, relieve local muscle spasm, promote local blood and lymph circulation, and improve the blood supply of the skin muscles. It is highly effective in relieving pain of the waist and back.

Instructions

❶ Press Yaoyan and Changqiang

Location

Yaoyan is located in a depression 10-13cm to the left side and right side of the fourth spinous process of the lumbar vertebra (Fig. 2-98); Changqiang is below the tip of the coccyx, in the middle between the tip of the coccyx and the anus (Fig. 2-99).

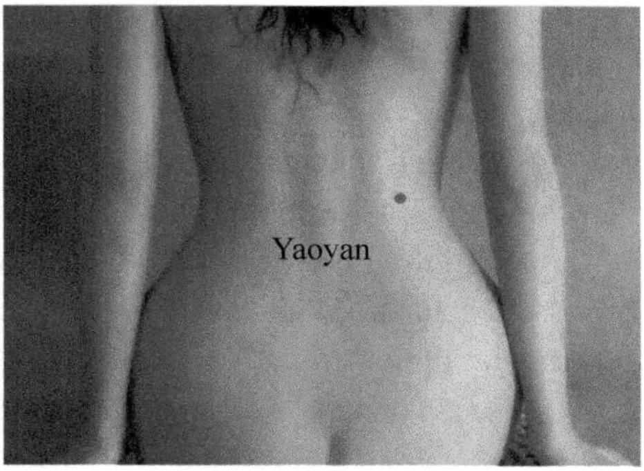

Fig. 2-98

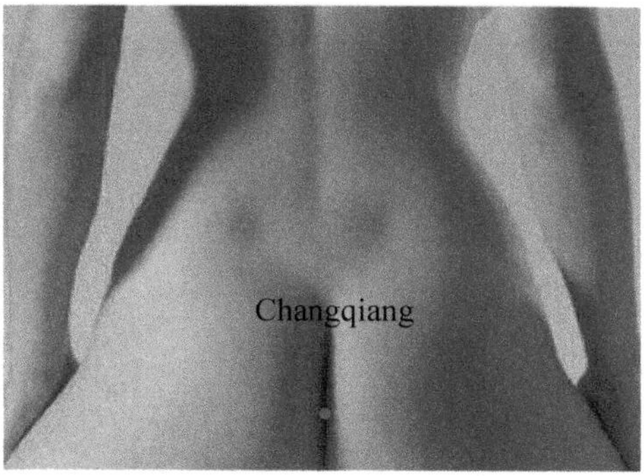

Fig. 2-99

Position

let your partner lie on his/her stomach on the bed.

Technique

Rub your hands until they get hot and press Yaoyan tightly. Seconds later rub downward to the coccyx (Changqiang). Rub once in the morning and once in the evening, 50-100 times each.

Then clench your fist lightly. Massage Yaoyan by revolving the front or back of your fist for 5 minutes.

❷ PressWeizhong

Location

Weizhong is located behind the knee joint, at the midpoint of the popliteal crease (Fig. 2-100).

Position

Let your partner lie on his/her stomach on the bed.

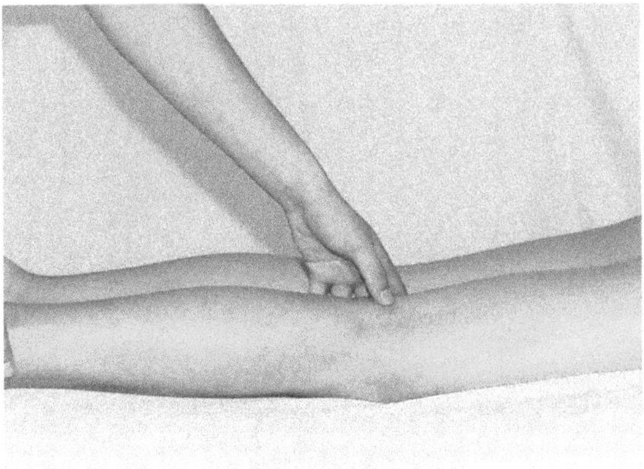

Fig. 2-100

Technique

Press Weizhong with two thumbs until your partner feels soreness. Press hardly and then press lightly. Press about 20 times, combined with flexion and extension of the knee.

❸ Press Ashi points

Location

The Ashi points are often located at the starting point and the ending point the of muscle, or where the pain is relatively shallow, as well as at the bulge of the muscle, or where the painful point is quite deep.

Position

Let your partner lie on his/her stomach on the bed.

Technique

Use the thumb pad, elbow tip or palm to press the affected area in a circular motion, gradually increase the pressure. Increase force gradually. Use the pad of your thumb to press the starting point and

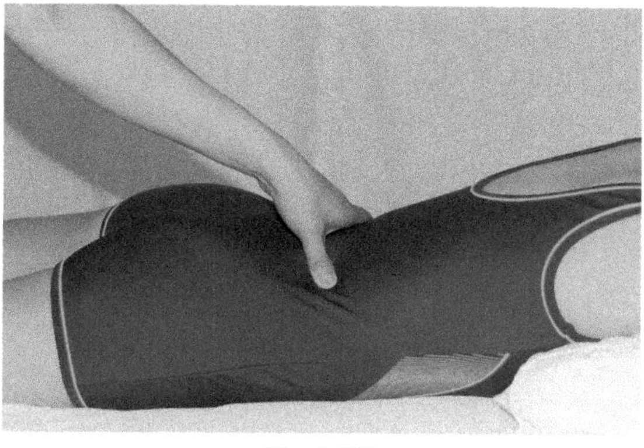

Fig. 2-101

the ending point of the muscle, or where the pain is relatively shallow (Ashi) ; use the elbow tip to press muscle bulge or where the painful point is quite deep (Ashi) (Fig. 2-101).

❹ Tapping method

This technique is similar to patting the back. Please let your partner lie on his/her stomach on the bed. Clench your fists and tap your partner's back from the thorax down the spine to the waist. You can also put the other hand onto your partner's lower back. Repeat the process (Fig. 2-102).

❺ Pinching method

Please let your partner lie on his/her stomach on the bed. Shape your thumb, forefinger, middle finger and ring finger like a plier and pinch your partner's waist (or back) muscles and tendons repeatedly. Pinch for 30-60 seconds at a time and repeat (Fig. 2-103).

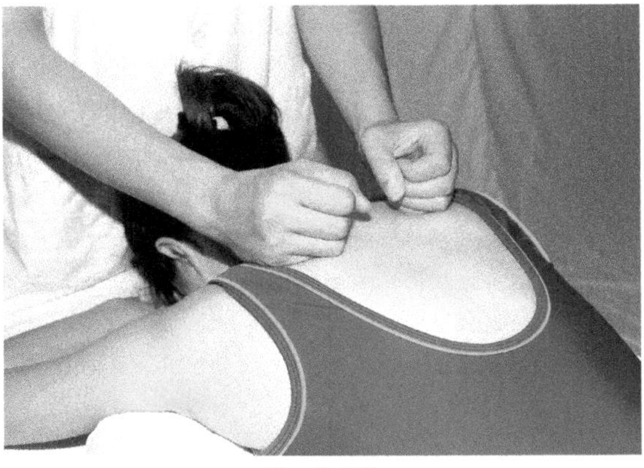

Fig. 2-102

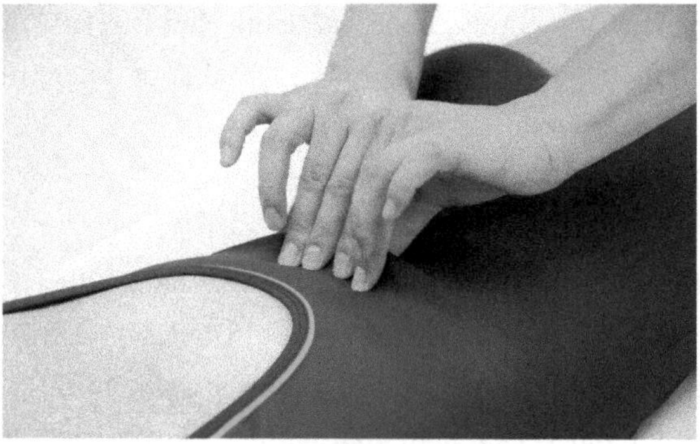

Fig. 2-103

Tips

1. Technique and intensity should be appropriate. On thick muscles, intensive techniques can be used; on shallow muscles, less intensive techniques should be used. Increase pressure and range gradually. Don't exceed the natural range of physiological movements.

2. Keep massage environment warm, and make sure that the patient is in a comfortable and relaxed position. Massage cannot be applied to patient who is too hungry or too full.

3. Safflower oil, essential balm, bonesetting liquid, and massage lotion can be used to strengthen the effects of massage. But as they can irritate the mucosa, they should not be used on the face, perineum and anus.

4. The best choice for massage is Guasha Oil or medicinal liquor. They can not only cure waist and back pain, but also relieve sore legs and other problems of the lower limbs.

Ankle Sprain

Stumbling or falling down when exercising on uneven ground, carrying heavy loads, walking down stairs, or walking on slopes can result in injured lateral ankle ligaments. Local effusion irritates peripheral nerves and causes pain and restriction of movement. This injury is called ankle sprain.

According to Chinese Medicine, when the ankle is injured, hemorrhage happens and causes swelling and pain.

Ankle sprain is common. Massage can relieve your partner's pain and enable him/her to walk again.

Instructions

1 Press the injured area of the ankle

Please let your partner sit on the bed or chair. Press the injured area with your thumb pad, and massage five times from the outer edge of the ankle via the outer edge of the shank to Yanglingquan, with Qiuxu, Xuanzhong and Yanglingquan as key points. Then push and press the injured area with your thumb, then push away from the area, in order to improve the blood circulation and dissipate blood stasis. You can do this until your partner feels soreness (Fig. 2-104).

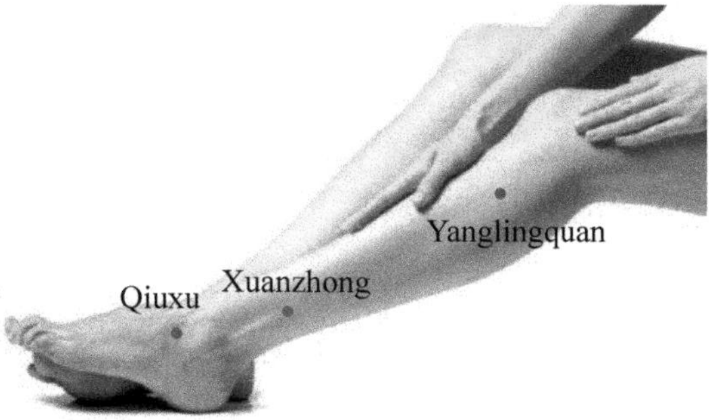

Fig. 2-104

❷ Shake and rotate the ankle joint

Please let your partner sit on the bed or chair and flex his/her injured limb. Squeeze the lower part in front of the tibia with one hand, fix the heel, and hold the front part of the foot with the other hand. Shake and rotate the ankle for 3 minutes (Fig. 2-105).

❸ Stretch back and flex foot sole

Please let your partner lie on the bed. Hold his/her heel with one hand and hold the foot sole with the other hand; pull the foot, stretch back, flex the foot sole, and shake the ankle joint (Fig. 2-106).

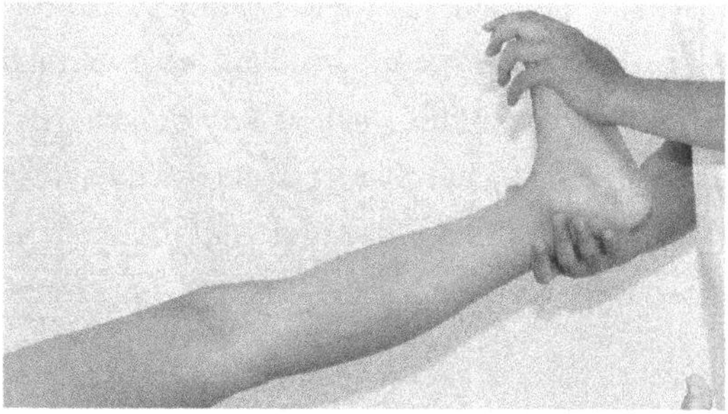

Fig. 2-105

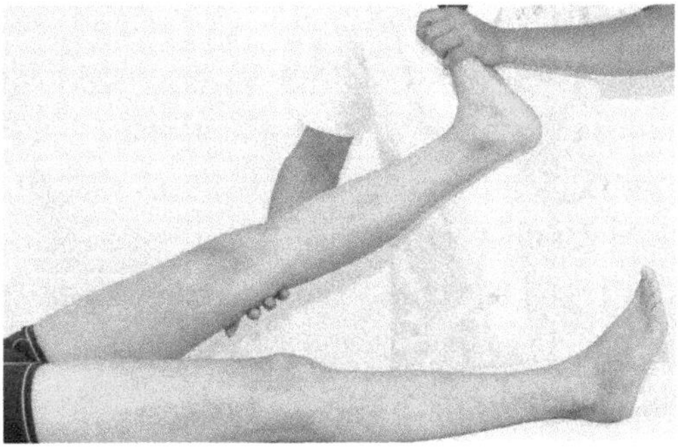

Fig. 2-106

❹ Hold and twist the toes, push and press the back of the foot

Please let your partner lie on the bed. Press his/her ankle with your left hand, and hold and twist his/her toes one by one with your thumb and forefinger. Then press and push the back of foot with your thumb pad until the skin turns red (Fig. 2-107).

❺ Pull and extend the ankle

Your partner will get a feeling of heat and have less pain when you

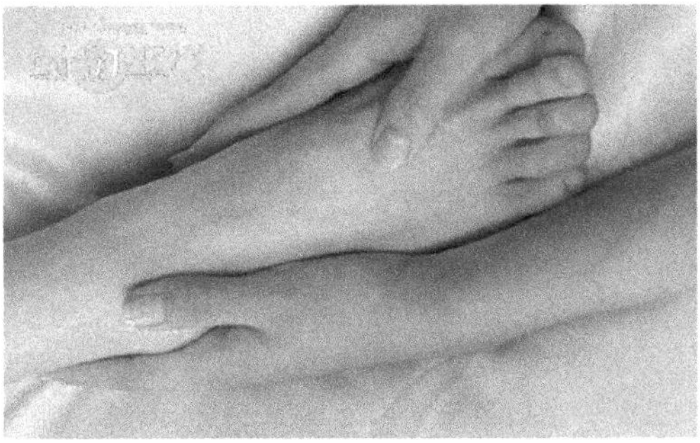

Fig. 2-107

finish the above methods. Then you can apply the key technique: pull the ankle and rotate it outward within a narrow range. Let your partner lie on the bed; hold his/her foot sole with one hand and fix the end of the ankle; press the injured area with the other hand, pull slowly and rotate it outward within a narrow range. Make sure you do it in a slow and gentle way. Then press Qiuxu and Yanglingquan until your partner feels soreness, and massage from the back of the foot via the ankle to the shank (Fig. 2-108).

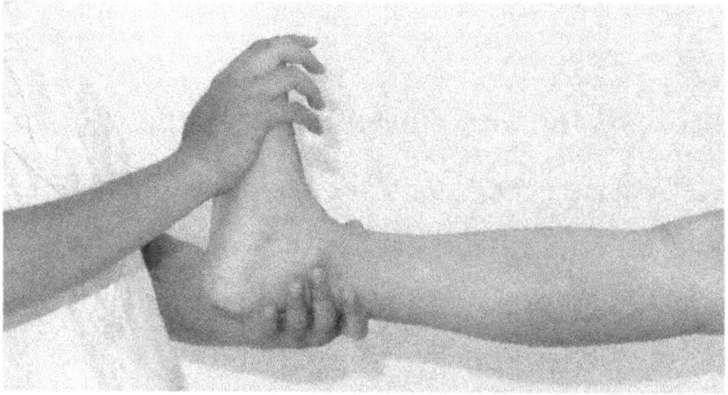

Fig. 2-108

Tips

1. Massage is not suggested within 24 hours after the ankle is hurt, otherwise it can aggravate hemorrhage.

2. If your partner has purple marks on the ankle, it is inadvisable to apply manipulative therapy or hot compresses immediately after injury. You should apply a cold compress first and apply manipulative therapy 24 hours later.

3. Massage gently.

4. Fix the injured part properly, keeping the foot from flexing inwards.

5. The effect will be better if a damp hot compress is applied.

✿ Lumbar Muscle Degeneration

Lumbar muscle degeneration, called functional back pain or waist and back myofascitis in medicine, refers to chronic impairment of lumbosacral muscles, fasciae and other soft tissues. This disease can be caused by bad posture leading to long-term waist muscle tension, uncured acute injury or getting soaked in cold and wet weather.

According to Chinese medicine, lumbar muscle degeneration is caused by cold-dampness, damp-heat, qi-stagnation and blood stasis, kidney deficiency and weakness, and injury by falling.

Massage can improve the kidneys and waist, expel wind and remove cold, relieving pain of the back and waist effectively.

Instructions

❶ Massage both sides of the waist

Let your partner lie on his/her stomach on the bed. Put your thumbs on both sides of the spine and the other fingers onto the sides of the waist. Use some strength to massage from waist to abdomen, repeat 30-50 times (Fig. 2-109).

❷ Rub the lumbosacral area

Let your partner lie on his/her stomach on the bed. Put your hand on both sides of the waist and rub it toward lumbosacral for 30-50

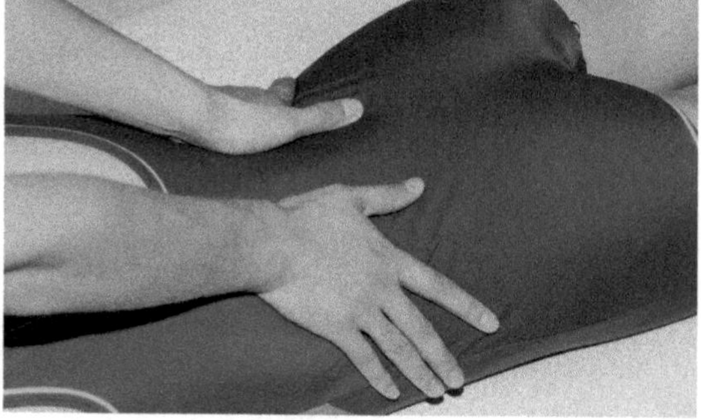

Fig. 2-109

times till your partner feels heat in waist (Fig. 2-110).

❸ Knock the lumbosacral area

Let your partner lie on his/her stomach on the bed. Clench your fists and knock on both sides of the lumbosacral area, repeat 30-50 times (Fig. 2-111).

❹ Massage around the navel

Let your partner lie on the bed. Put one of your palms onto the

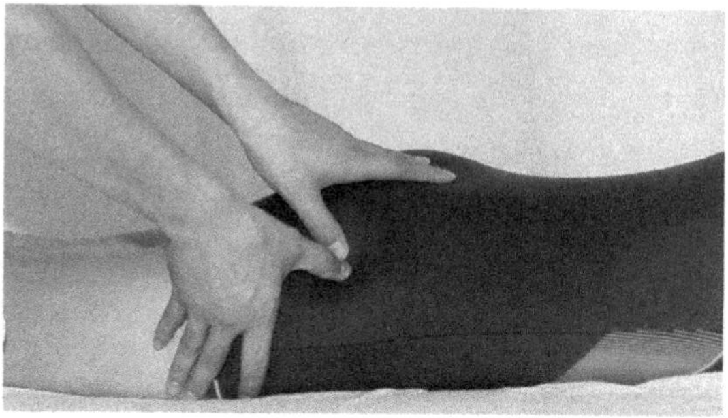

Fig. 2-110

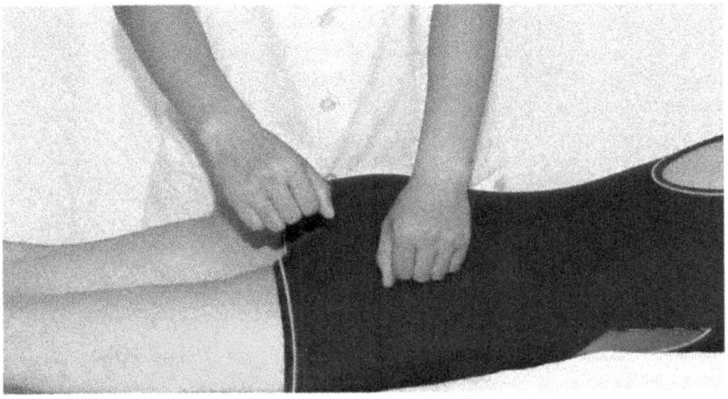

Fig. 2-111

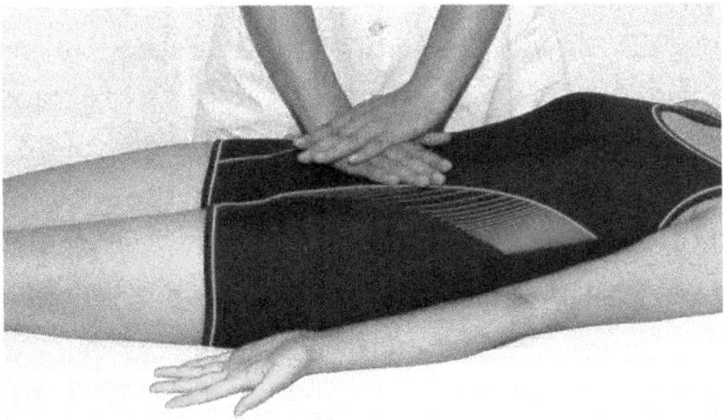

Fig. 2-112

point 2 inches above your partner's navel and the other palm onto the back of the first hand. Then use some strength to massage around the navel for 30-50 circles (Fig. 2-112).

Tips

You best apply the described massage methods twice a day, once in the morning and once in the evening. Long-time practice will bring about good effects.

Cerebral Stroke Sequelae

Cerebral stroke, also called cerebral apoplexy or cerebrovascular accident, presents with lack of blood in the brain and hemorrhagic injury as main symptoms. The onset is rapid and acute, it develops fast like the unpredictable wind, so it is called "wind stroke" in Chinese medicine. When a blood vessel of the brain gets injured, the brain tissue becomes short of blood, gets pressed and pushed by hematoma or cerebral edema. When brain tissue gets damaged, brain functions are also impaired; for example, endocyst hemorrhage may cause contralateral hemiplegia left-sided hemorrhage may lead to aphasia; after the acute period, hemiplegia may become spastic with the upper limbs flexed and adducted and the lower limbs extended. Furthermore, there is a tendon hyperreflexia and the motor abilities may recover. As time goes by, hemiplegic limbs can gradually move again. The lower limbs recover earlier than the upper limbs; proximal parts recover better than distal ones; the last and most difficult to recover are the fine finger movements.

According to Chinese Medicine, cerebral stroke sequelae are mainly caused by weakness of qi, stagnation of blood, blockage of veins, deficiency of kidneys and liver, deficiency of essence and blood, or bad nourishing of muscles and bones after stroke.

Brain stroke presents with a high rate of fatality and disability. Serious stroke can be life-threatening. A patient who survives after treatment in hospital may suffer impediment in movement, feeling and language. It takes a long time to recover; therefore more attention should be paid in daily care. Massage is a simple and effective treatment which clears and activates the channels and collaterals, keeping the situation from worsening.

Instructions

❶ Roll fingers (toes)

Let your partner lie on the bed. Roll each finger and toe of his/her paralyzed hands and feet gently, from thumb (big toe) to little finger (little toe). Every side of the fingers or toes should be rolled. This method takes 20 minutes. It helps to improve peripheral blood circulation, prevents muscles from withering and promotes the recovery of nerves (Fig. 2-113).

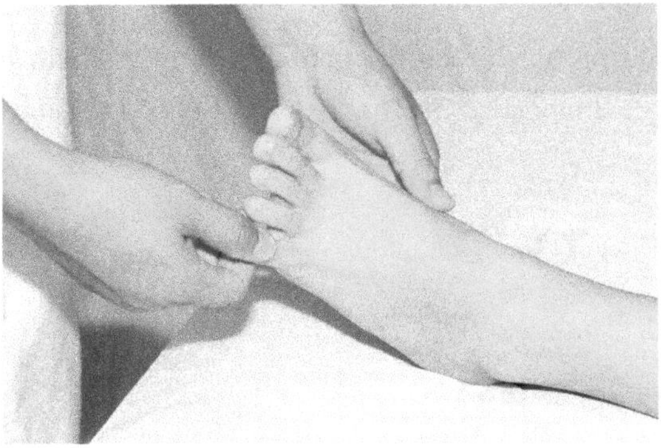

Fig. 2-113

❷ Massage the limbs

Let your partner lie on the bed. Massage the paralyzed limbs softly, especially the muscles of the outside of arms and legs. Stroke patients usually suffer from muscle atrophy on the outer and frontal sides of the limbs. Massaging these muscles can prevent atrophy effectively (Fig. 2-114).

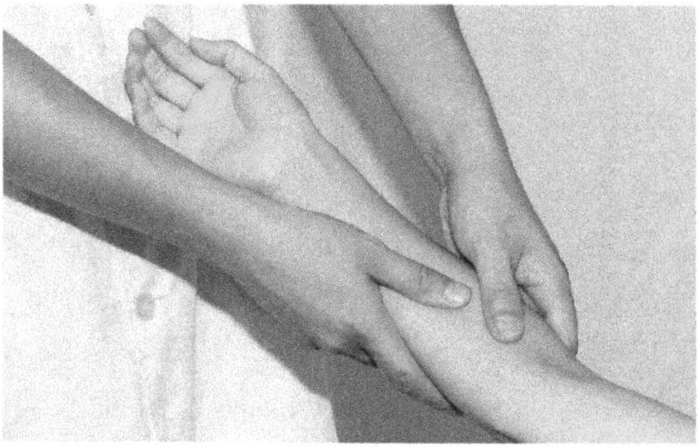

Fig. 2-114

❸ Press Hegu, Quchi, Zusanli and Sanyinjiao

Let your partner lie on the bed or sit on the chair. Press Hegu (Fig. 2-115), Quchi (Fig. 2-116), Zusanli (Fig. 2-117) and Sanyinjiao

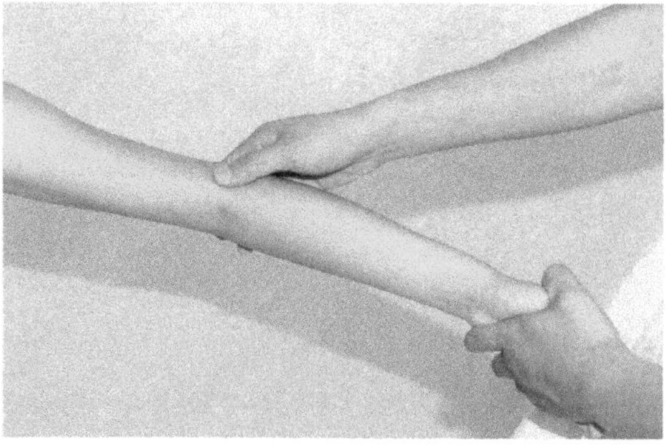

Fig. 2-115

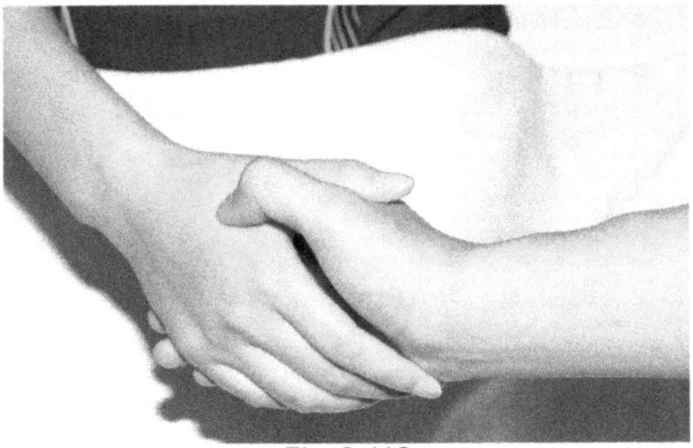

Fig. 2-116

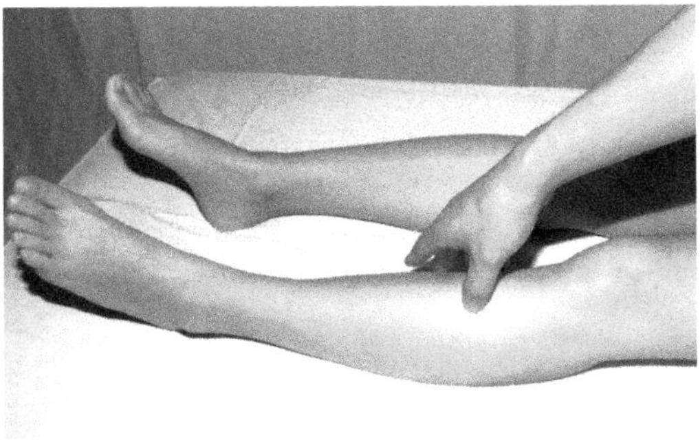

Fig. 2-117

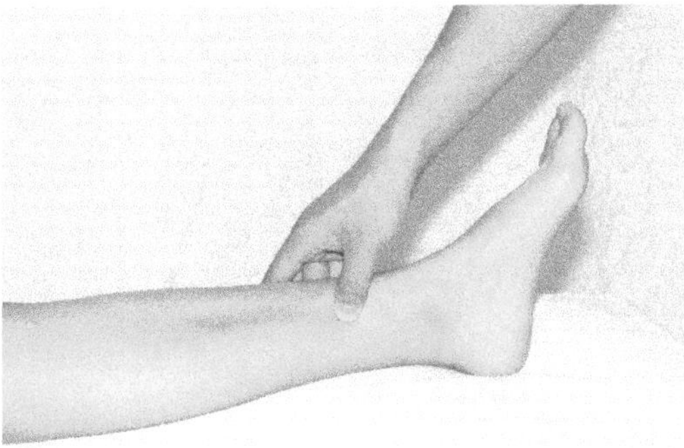

Fig. 2-118

(Fig. 2-118) with thumb for 1 minute each. This has the effect of invigorating qi and blood as well as clearing and activating the channels and collaterals.

❹ Massage the movable joints

Let your partner lie on the bed. Move the joints of the limbs starting at the most distal ones. Use appropriate strength, watch out not injure the joints or hurt your partner. Exercise the joints of fingers, palm and wrist first, then exercise elbow and shoulder joints exercise joints of toes and ankle before exercising joints of knee and hip. Remember to often practice lifting and stretching the thigh (Fig. 2-119).

❺ Help your partner to move the joint by him/herself

After you exercise your partner's paralyzed limb joint, you can help him/her to exercise the "paralyzed hand" with his/her own

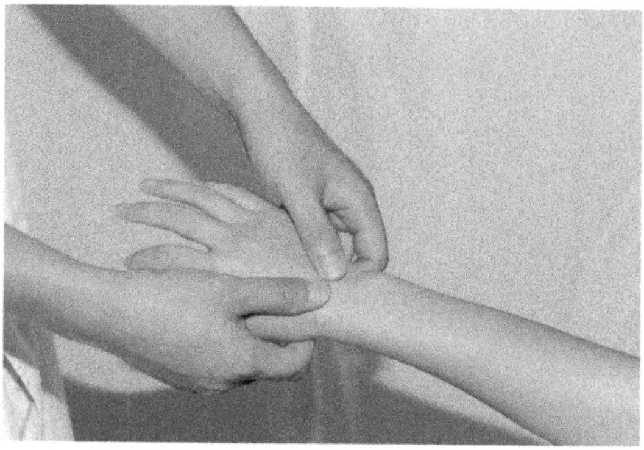

Fig. 2-119

"healthy hand". For example, let your partner lie on the bed and lift his/her arm softly.

Tips

1. Start massaging as soon as you can; generally speaking, as long as the patient's situation and vital signs (body temperature, breath, pulse, and blood pressure) are stable, massage can be applied.

2. As stroke can reduce the range of movement, most patients are not enthusiastic about exercising. Therefore, it is necessary to urge and assist your partner to exercise. Exercise in an appropriate way in order not to damage the muscles and joints and combine with medicinal therapy.

3. Apart from using the mentioned methods, you can also encourage and help your partner to do some "housework". You can start with pointing at a cup, holding it, taking up a pen and using chopsticks. When your partner is able to complete these movements, you can help him/her to exercise having a meal, dressing him/herself, pouring water, and then drawing a picture, writing, etc.

Chronic Prostatitis

Chronic prostatitis can be divided into chronic bacterial prostatitis and chronic nonbacterial prostatitis. The former one is caused by bacterial infection and the latter one is caused by unknown reasons which may be related with urinary dysfunction, neuroendocrine factors, psychological factors and pelvic factors. It mainly manifests with pelvic girdle pain, which can be felt in the area of the perineum, the perianal, urethra, pubis and the lumbosacral area. There can be urinary symptoms like urgent, frequent or painful urination and nocturia. As the pain becomes chronic, the patient's living quality will be influenced and sexual dysfunction, anxiousness, depression, insomnia and hypomnesia can occur.

According to Chinese medicine, prostatitis can be regarded as effulgent fire, stagnation due to dampness-heat, stasis of qi and blood and kidney deficiency of yin and yang.

Massage can directly stimulate and enhance the functions of the prostate while increasing the urination to assist recovery. Massage can significantly improve chronic prostatitis.

Instructions

❶ Press "The Inner Triangle"

"The Inner Triangle" refers to a triangle area or a trapezoid area of the male lower abdomen and perineum. Two sides of the triangle are the lymph glands of the higher thigh, with the position of Jimai, Chongmen and Fushe, while the lower side of the triangle is at the symphysis. This position is significant for both male and female. Generally, it is not easy to exercise The Inner Triangle in daily life. Due to the sedentary lifestyle, the blood circulation is not smooth and male and female reproductive diseases occur, especially prostate problems.

During massage, your partner can lie on the bed. Use some strength to press the three edge points of The Inner Triangle, putting your forefinger, middle finger and fourth finger together. You might feel the unevenness of the lymph glands (Fig. 2-120).

❷ Press Taichong, Gongsun, Taixi, Sanyinjiao, Yinlingquan

Location

Taichong is located on the dorsum of the foot, in a depression distal to the junction of the first and second metatarsal bones (Fig.

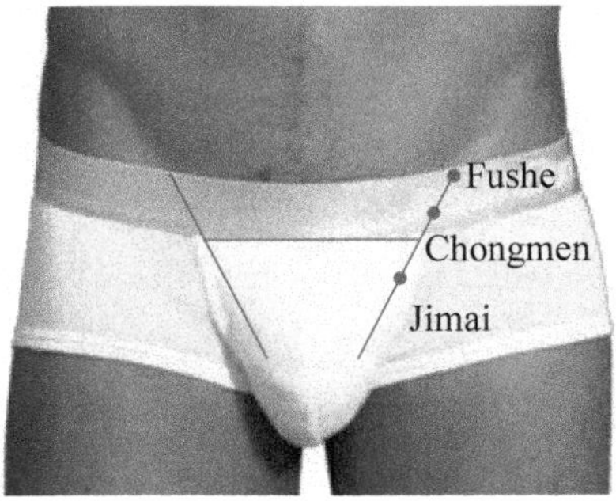

Fig. 2-120

2-121) Gongsun is on the inner side of the foot, in a depression distal to the first metatarsal. Taixi is in between the malleolus medialis and the Achilles tendon. Sanyinjiao is one hand-width above the tip of the malleolus medialis behind the Tibia. Yinlingquan is located at the inside of the knee, in a depression inferior and posterior to the medial condyle of the tibia (Fig. 2-122).

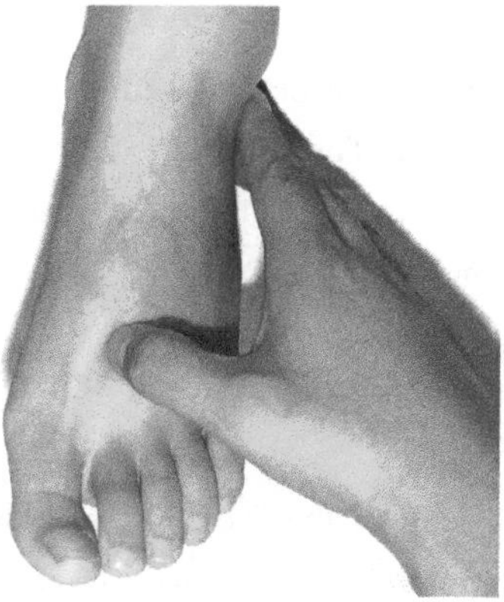

Fig. 2-121

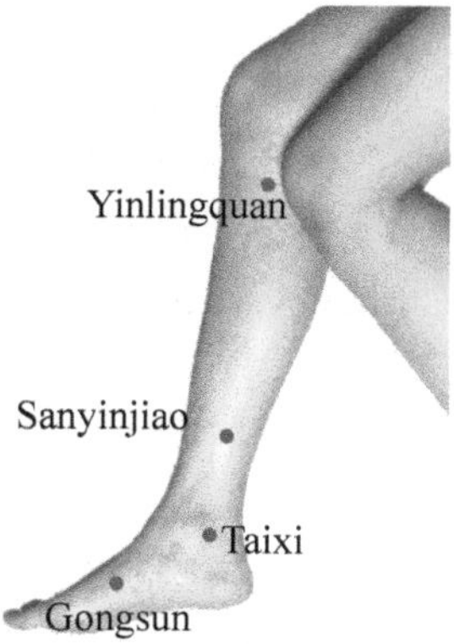

Fig. 2-122

Position

Let your partner lie on the bed

Technique

Press Taichong, Gongsun, Taixi, Sanyinjiao, Yinlingquan. Usually, there will be effects with just pressing once and the problem can be cured within 20 days of treatment.

Tips

1. Many people are worried about the pain felt during massage or the knotty tissues. Slowly increase the pressure as much as your partner feels is bearable, the area will get smoother with time and the pain will slowly vanish.

2. The most obvious result is a smoother urination.

3. When you press Qugu (CV2), your partner might get an erection, don't worry about it, as it means that the blood circulation gets going.

Dysmenorrhea

Dysmenorrhea refers to the spasmodic pain in the lower abdomen that can occur around menstruation and affect daily life and the general well-being.

According to Chinese medicine, there are two reasons of dysmenorrhea. One reason is pain from deficiency, caused by deficiency of qi and blood or depletion of liver and kidneys. The other reason is stagnation leading to pain, which is caused by stagnant movement of Qi and blood.

Massage can help strengthen the liver qi and relieve the pain, it is a good prevention and treatment method.

Instructions

❶ Massage the lower abdomen

Let your partner lie on the bed. Put both of your hands onto the middle of the area between the navel and genitalia. Put pressure onto the abdomen and slowly massage it with a frequency of 10 times per minute until you can feel the heat , which takes about 5 minutes (Fig. 2-123).

❷ Press Sanyinjiao and Taichong

Location

Sanyinjiao is one hand-width above the tip of the malleolus medialis behind the Tibia (Fig. 2-124). Taichong is located on the

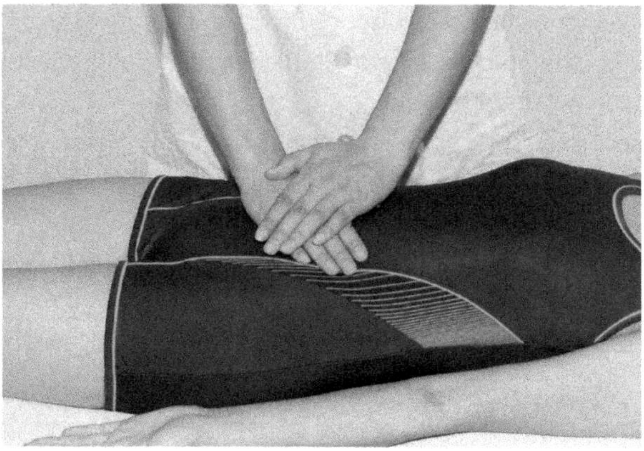

Fig. 2-123

dorsum of the foot, in a depression distal to the junction of the first and second metatarsal bones (Fig. 2-125).

Location

Let your partner lie on the bed.

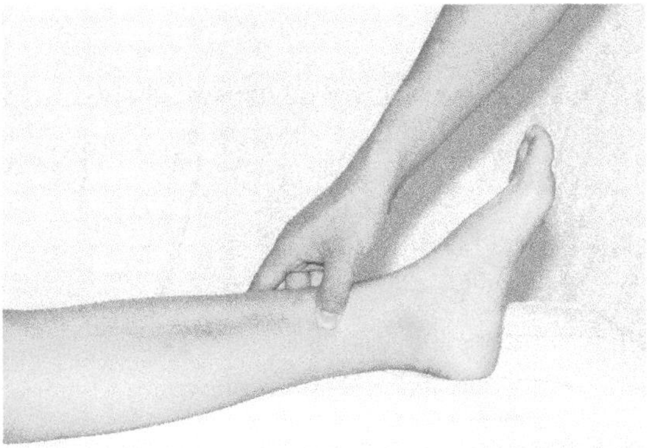

Fig. 2-124

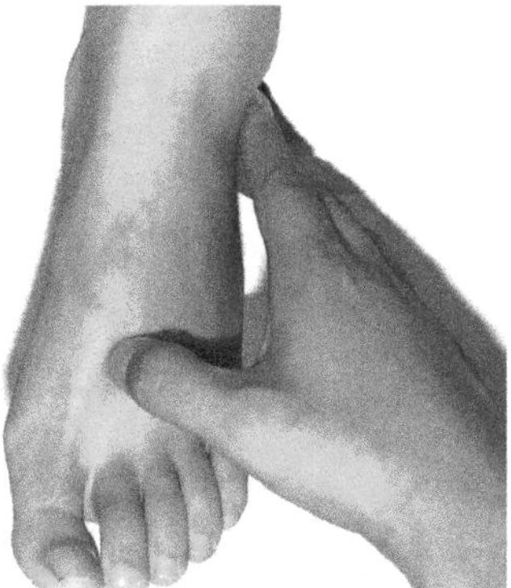

Fig. 2-125

Technique

Press Sanyinjiao with the thumb until your partner can feel some soreness of the muscle. Wait for a minute, then press Taichong for one more minute.

❸ Press Zigong

Location

Zigong is located on the lower abdomen, about 13 cm below the navel and 10 cm lateral to the median line (Fig. 2-126).

Position

Let your partner lie on the bed.

Technique

Use both forefingers and middle fingers to put pressure on Zigong. Slowly rub the point for about five minutes until your partner gets a sore and hot feeling.

❹ Rolling Taichong

Location

Taichong is located on the dorsum of the foot, in a depression

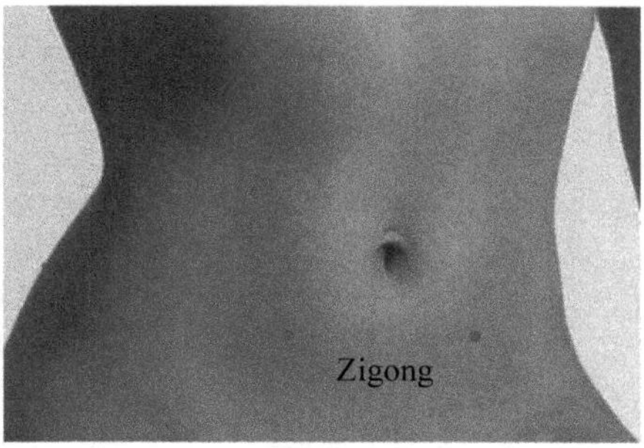

Fig. 2-126

distal to the junction of the first and second metatarsal bones (Fig. 2-127).

Position

Let your partner lie on the bed.

Technique

Press Taichong on the right side with the left thumb until it feels sore. 1 minute later, press Taichong on the left side with the right thumb for another minute.

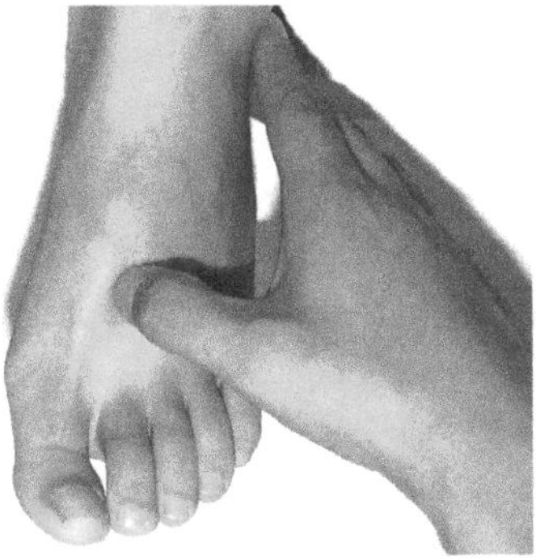

Fig. 2-127

Tips

1. The treatment of dysmenorrheal generally focuses on the period of 5-7 days before menstruation. Pressing the points can prevent dysmenorrhea.

2. The goal of the massage is to help the blood descending. So use this method when you feel pain in the lower abdomen and the lumbosacral area. If it is done properly, the menstruation can start 1-2 days earlier and the pain will be released with it.

Abnormal Leucorrhea

Leucorrhea refers to the white colored vaginal secretion of a physically mature female. Under normal circumstances, the small amount of white odorless leucorrhea shows that her spleen and kidneys are healthy. The leucorrhea can help to moisten the vagina and prevent bacterial infections. Before and after the menstruation, the amount of leucorrhea will slightly increase, which is physiologically normal. If the quantity is large, the consistency too thick or too thin, or if it is coloured, has a smell with local irritation or general symptoms, then it becomes pathological and is called profuse discharge.

According to Chinese medicine, abnormal leucorrhea is mainly caused by a deficient spleen failing to transport, renal deficient kidneys failing to consolidate, accumulation of damp heat and restraint of the belt vessel.

Massage can help to replenish the spleen, get rid of dampness and stop the leucorrhea with better effects than drug therapy. There are no side effects and it benefits the whole reproductive system.

Instructions

❶ Rub and vibrate the lower abdomen

Let your partner lie on the bed and use your palm to rub the lower abdomen in a clockwise and anticlockwise direction for 1-2 minutes respectively. The manipulation should be deep and gentle. Then vibrate the abdomen with the palm for 1-2 minutes (Fig. 2-128).

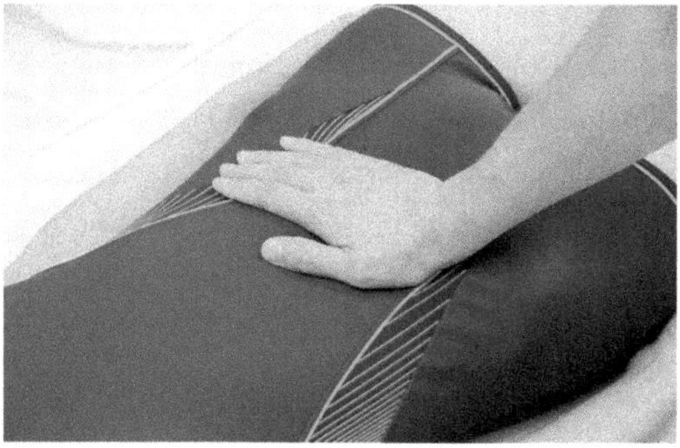

Fig. 2-128

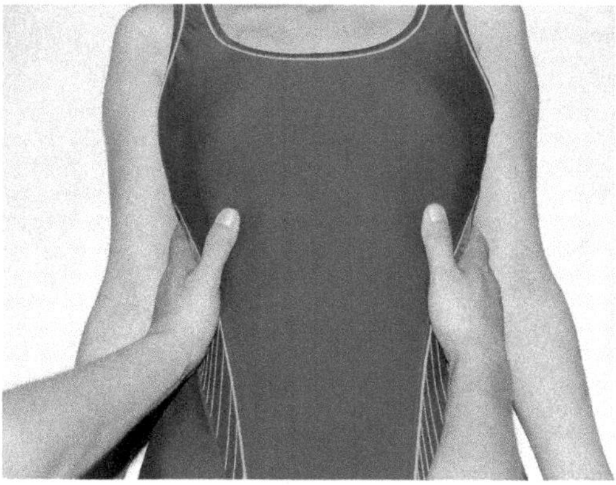

Fig. 2-129

❷ Massage the waist and abdomen

Let your partner lie on the bed, hold your partner's waist with both hands, massage down the back and rub towards the lower abdomen. Then rub along the groin to the symphysis, repeat 10 to 15 times (Fig. 2-129).

❸ Rub Haixue and press Yinlingquan and Sanyinjiao

Location

Haixue is about 6.5 cm above the medial corner of the patella, on the bulge of the quadriceps (Fig. 2-130). Yinlingquan is located at the inside of the knee, in a depression inferior and posterior to the medial condyle of the tibia. Sanyinjiao is located on the medial side of the calf, a hand-width above the tip of the inner ankle bone (Fig. 2-132).

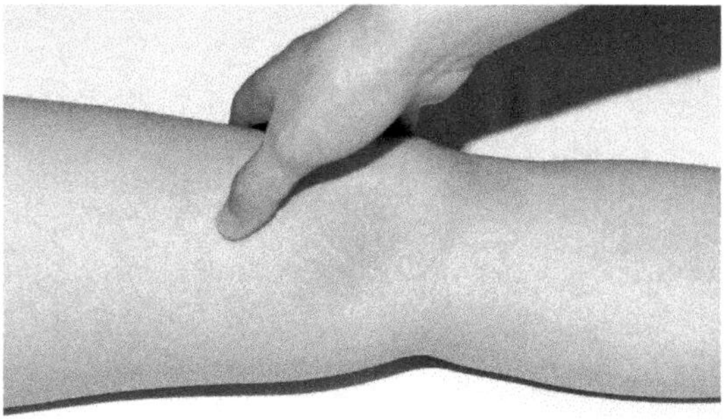

Fig. 2-130

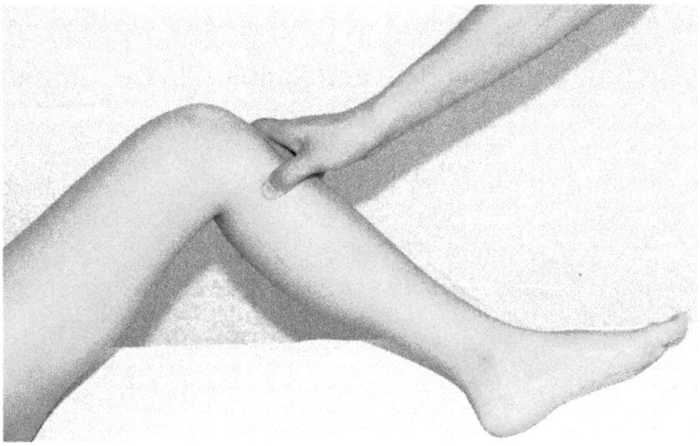

Fig. 2-131

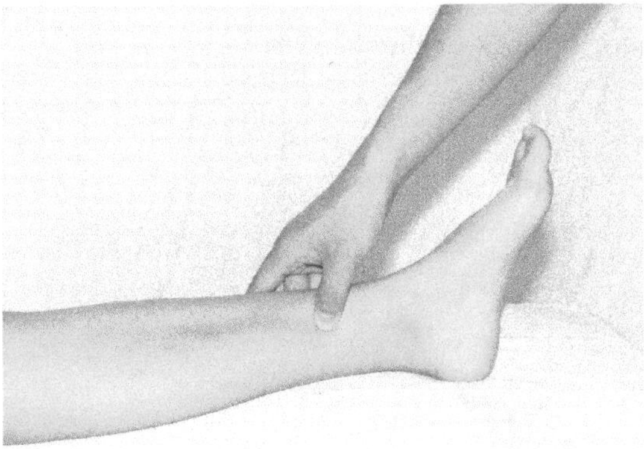

Fig. 2-132

Location

Let your partner lie on the bed.

Technique

Put both of your thumbs on Haixue and put the other fingers on the muscles of the knee, press and rub the area for 20 minutes. After this, press and pluck Yinlingquan and Sanyinjiao for 1 minute.

❹ Rub Baliao and press Changqiang

Location

Baliao are located on the sacral vertebrae, they are also named Shangliao, Ciliao, Zhongliao and Xialiao. There are eight points altogether in the 1st, 2nd, 3rd and 4th sacral foramen, called "Baxue" (Fig. 2-133); Changqiang is below the tip of the coccyx, in the middle between the tip of the coccyx and the anus (Fig. 2-134).

Position

Let your partner lie on the stomach.

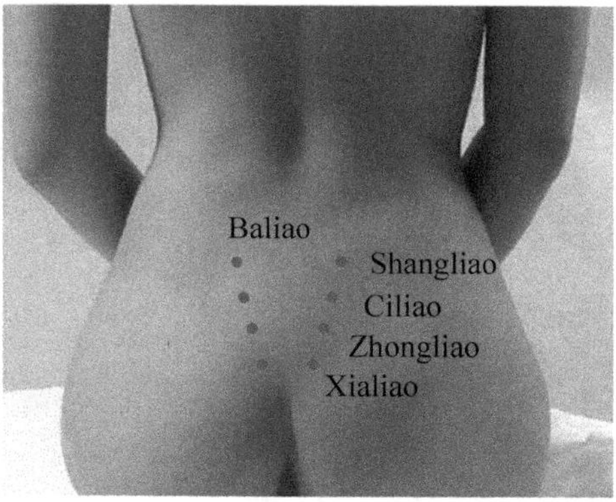

Fig. 2-133

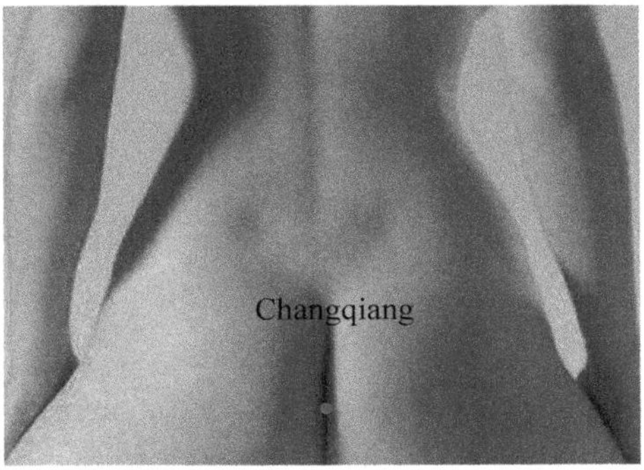

Fig. 2-134

Technique

Rub "Baxue" on the lumbosacral area. Repeat the procedure until your partner can feel the heat; press Changqiang with both forefingers and middle fingers, repeat 7-10 times.

Tips

Keep rubbing once a day. Abstain from sex for a while, until the symptoms get better.

✿ Menopausal Syndrome

Menopausal Syndrome refers to the period from a child-bearing age to old age. Since there are changes in the sexual glands, functional disturbances of the vegetative nerve system can occur. The menopausal syndrome can be seen after the decline of ovarian functions, and correspondingly, sex hormones will decrease. Then the cerebral cortex and vegetative nerve functions will be disturbed. This mainly reflects in paroxysmal facial flush, headache, head distention, hypomnesis, emotional tension, insomnia, hypodynamia, palpitations, disorders of blood pressure, soreness of the waist, frequent urination, hyposexuality and osteoporosis.

According to Chinese medicine, during the female menopause, the kidney qi gradually fades. The penetrating and conception vessels are getting weak; the essence and blood are becoming deficient; the reproductive functions are gradually lost and the organ functions are declining, leading to a disharmony of yin and yang.

Massage can help to harmonize yin and yang, nourish the mind and relieve discomfort to a great extent.

Instructions

❶ Massage the abdomen

Let your partner lie on the bed. Please overlap your hands on the belly and massage 300-500 times both clockwise and anticlockwise until your partner can feel the heat (Fig. 2-135).

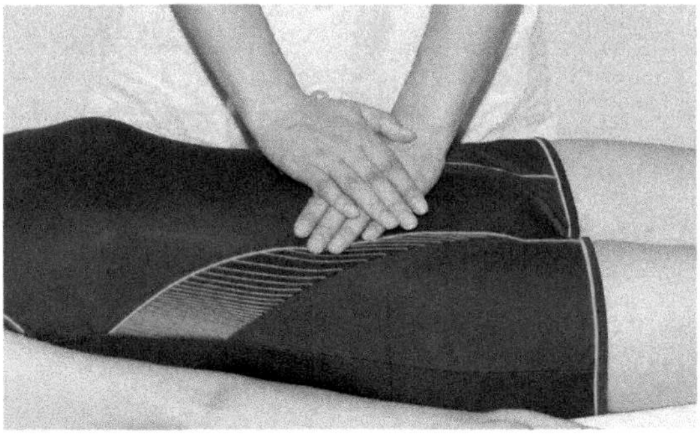

Fig. 2-135

❷ Press Qihai and Guanyuan

Location

Qihai is on the middle line of the lower abdomen, about 5cm below the navel; Guanyuan is on the middle line of the lower abdomen, about 10cm below the navel (Fig. 2-136).

Position

Let your partner lie on the belly.

Technique

Press Qiahai and Guanyuan with the thumb, repeat 100-200 times

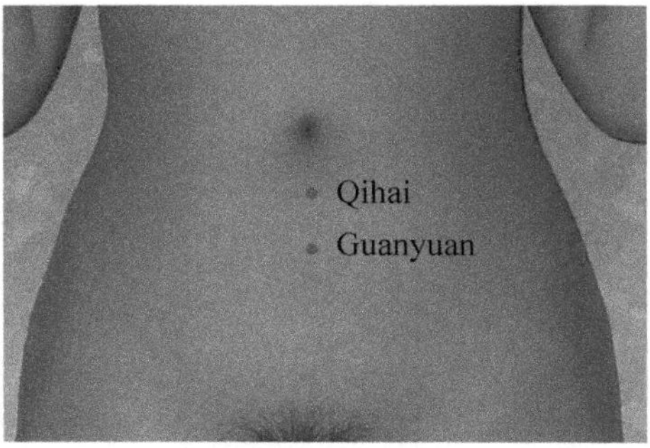

Fig. 2-136

until your partner can feel soreness and swelling.

❸ Push and press Taiyang and Guanyuan

Location

Taiyang is located on the forehead in between the two brows; Taiyang is located in a depression about one finger-width posterior to the lateral end of the eyebrow and the outer canthus (Fig. 2-137).

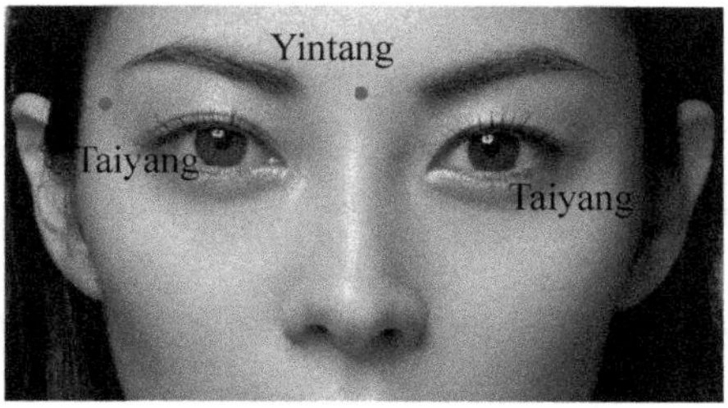

Fig. 2-137

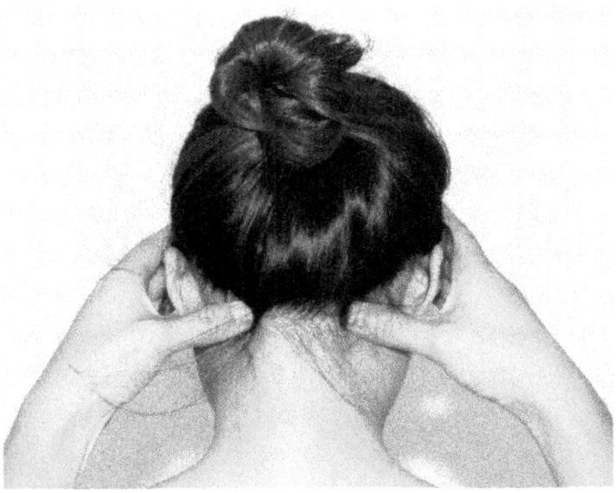

Fig. 2-138

Position

Let your partner sit straight.

Technique

Push and press from Yintang to Taiyang with your forefinger, middle finger and ring finger, repeat 5-10 times.

❹ Press Fengchi

Location

Fengchi is located below the occipital bone on the neck, in a depression between sternocleidomastoid and trapezius (Fig. 2-138).

Position

Let your partner sit straight.

Technique

Press Fengchi with the middle finger, repeat 100-200 times

❺ Press Danzhong

Location

Danzhong is on the median line, in between the nipples (Fig. 2-139).

Position

Let your partner lie on the bed.

Technique

Press Danzhong for 100-200 times.

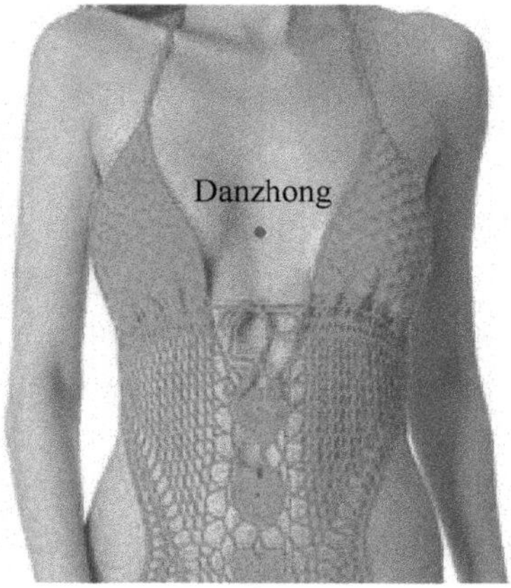

Fig. 2-139

Tips

1. Massage 1-2 times a day.

2. The results will be even better if combined with exercises like walking or jogging.

3. Please see a doctor if the symptoms get more serious.

Chronic Hyperplasia of Mammary Glands

Hyperplasia of the mammary glands is a common female breast disease. Although it usually is not a life-threatening disease, the distending pain in the breast is still very disturbing. Mild hyperplasia of the mammary glands often manifests periodically; it feels worse before menstruation and then it gets better after the period has started. Women of older age who have never breast-fed or who have depression are more prone to get this ailment.

According to Chinese medicine, hyperplasia of mammary glands is mostly related to disorders of organ functions and qi-blood disharmony. There is a saying that organ function disorders are mostly caused by disharmony of liver and spleen, especially affecting the people whose spleen is weak or who eat too much spicy and greasy food, which can damage the spleen and cause disorders. It can also be caused by emotional depression and bad temper; all the emotional factors can affect the controlling function of the liver and lead to the stagnation of phlegm-dampness and the accumulation of qi and blood. This can lead to mammary masses.

It is easy to massage the breast and treat hyperplasia of the mammary glands. And it works very well.

Instructions

❶ Massage the breast

Please let your partner lie on the bed. Put a little paraffin or olive oil on one side of the breast and then gently push and massage the breasts in the direction of the nipples, repeat 50-100 times.

❷ Press the breast

Please let your partner sit or lie on the bed. Press firm but gently with the thenar or hypothenar of the palm. Then knead the area around the nipple with your palm until any hard masses disappear, repeat 50-100 times.

❸ Pinch the breast

Please let your partner sit or lie on the bed. Then, hold your

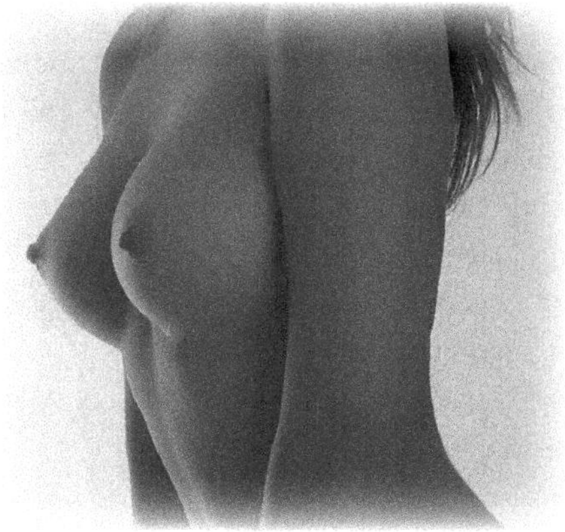

Fig. 2-140

partner's breasts and gently pinch the lateral sides of the breasts for 10-15 times, alternately loose and tight. Finally pull the nipples several times to expand milk ducts.

❹ Vibrate the breast

Please let your partner sit or lie on the bed. Vibrate and push the breast from the knotty parts of the breast to the nipples with your right hypothenar for 3-5 times, repeat until your partner locally feels some heat (Fig. 2-140).

Tips

1. The massage for hyperplasia of mammary glands is just relieving it, please go to see a doctor to cure the hyperplasia.

2. Please pay attention to the direction, strength, sequence and frequency.

3. Please be aware that you will need long-term practice of the methods mentioned to move away the hyperplasia.

Vomiting during Pregnancy

Vomiting during pregnancy refers to a normal physical reaction in pregnancy. During this period, a woman's gastric acid and digestive enzymes decrease, influencing the normal digesting function. She will feel dizzy, nauseous, have a lack of appetite or even vomit.

According to Chinese medicine, pregnancy vomiting is caused by various factors, for example damp-heat, deficient cold and the failure of descending of stomach-qi. Different factors will all lead to disharmony of the middle energizer and adverse rising of stomach qi. All these causes result in vomiting.

Under the normal circumstances, please find your doctor if there is some intense symptoms. Mild vomiting will not affect the woman's health, but the partner can help to relief the symptoms.

Instructions

❶ Push the upper abdomen

Please let your partner lie on the bed. Push the upper abdomen gently with the whole palm in an anticlockwise direction, repeat 3-5 minutes per day (Fig. 2-141).

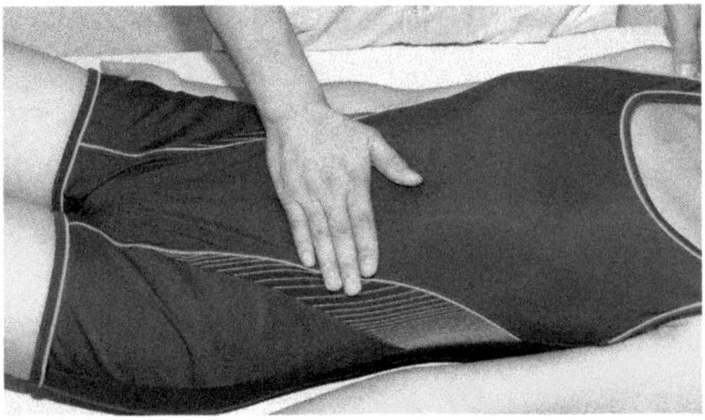

Fig. 2-141

❷ Press Neiguan and Zusanli

Location

Spread your partner's palm. Then find the Neiyuan 6.5 cm above the inside of the wrist, in between the tendons (Fig. 2-142); Zusanli is located at about 6.5 cm below the depression on the outer side of the

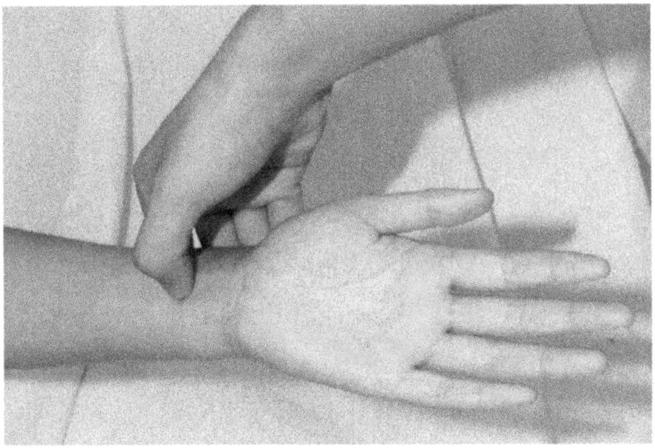

Fig. 2-142

knee, about one finger-width lateral to the crest of the tibia (Fig. 2-143).

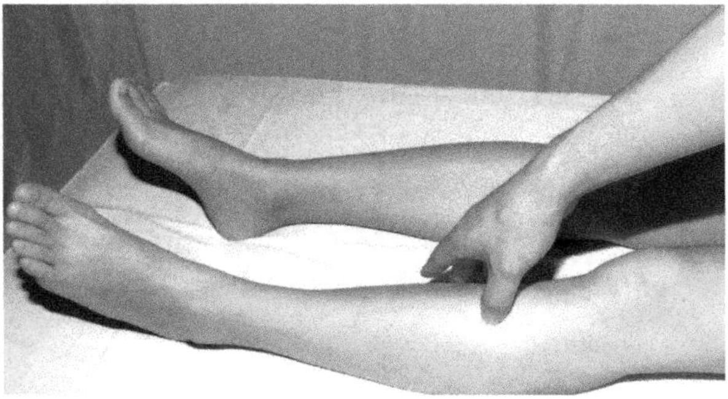

Fig. 2-143

Position

Let your partner sit straight.

Technique

Please rub the right Neiguan with your left forefinger and middle finger, and then change to the other hand for 20-30 times respectively; Press Zusanli with both thumbs, repeat 20-30 times.

❸ Rub Chongyang, Taibai and Shangyang

Location

Chongyang is located on the top of the foot where you can feel the pulsation of the artery (Fig. 2-144). Taibai is on the inner side of the foot, in a depression under the first metatarsal (Fig. 2-145). Shangyang is just next to the radial angle of the index finger's nail (Fig. 2-146).

Position

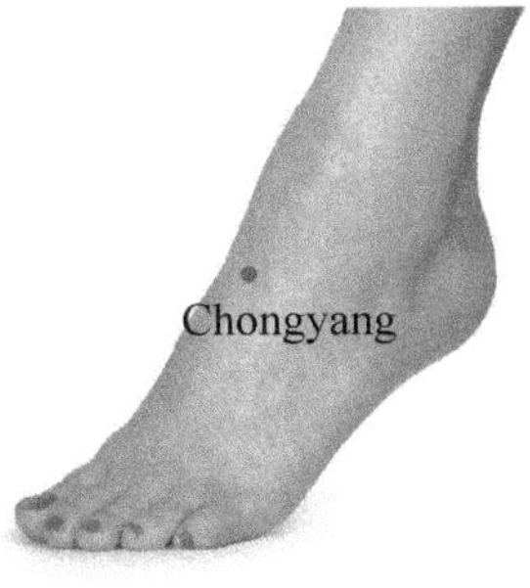

Fig. 2-144

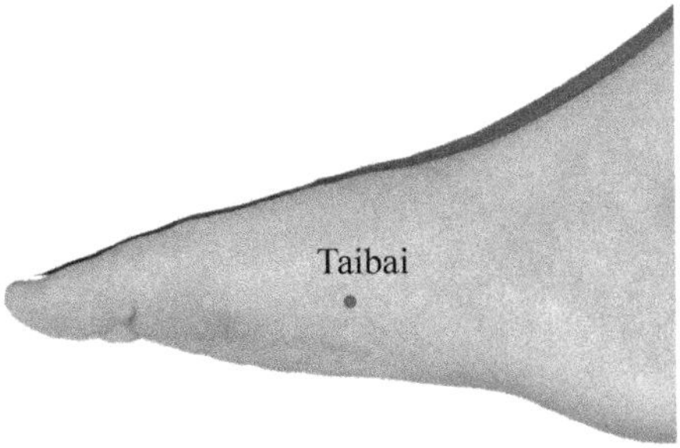

Fig. 2-145

Please let your partner sit straight with the feet evenly on the ground.

Technique

Kneel down in front of your partner and put your partner's feet on your knees. Then rub Chongyang and Taibai for 10 minutes

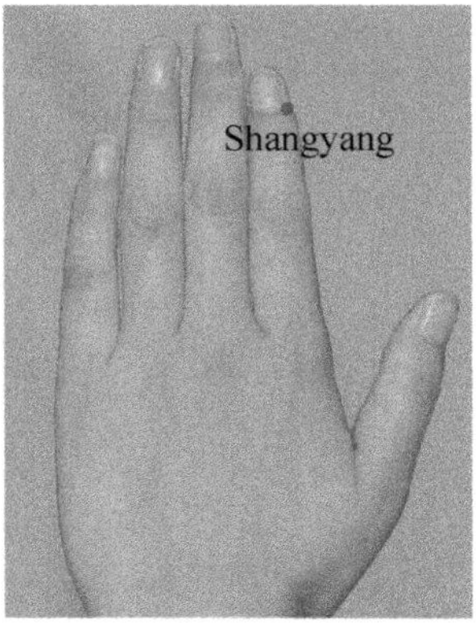

Fig. 2-146

respectively; Then rub Shangyang for 3-5 minutes per day.

Tips

1. Massage the feet gently, don't use heavy pressure.

2. You can do the first technique if the vomiting is not serious; if it is heavy, you can use the third technique.

Inadequate Secretion of Milk

The secretion of milk is related to many factors such as mental, emotional and nutritional factors. Any mental irritation such as anxiousness, panic, worries, fright or sorrow will decrease the secretion. Inadequate secretion of milk refers to the inability of breast-feeding the baby properly. Reasons for this may be poor development of the mammary glands or emotional instability. Other factors such as infection, diarrhea, loose stool and blockage of the glands can also lead to inadequate secretion.

According to Chinese medicine, inadequate secretion of milk can be divided into deficiency and excess. Deficiency results in deficient blood and qi and a lack of resource for milk; excess results in stagnation of liver qi or stasis of blood leading to a blockage of the milk delivery.

Massage can be done at home. It can help supplementing qi and nourishing blood, assist the free flow of the liver, control the emotions and activate the collaterals. All the methods can help with the milk secretion.

Instructions

❶ Massage the breast

Let your partner sit or lie on the bed. Please massage the breast gently for 1-3 minutes.

❷ Rub the breast

Let your partner sit and lie on the bed. Please rub the breast 10-20 times with your fingers and then vibrate the breast for 1-3 minutes (Fig. 2-147).

❸ Press Rugen

Location

Rugen locates under the nipple and beside the breast root, 13cm

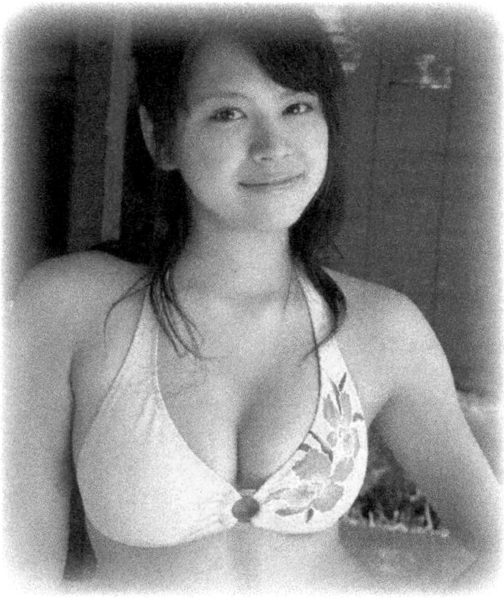

Fig. 2-147

away from the middle line. There is one point on each breast (Fig. 2-148).

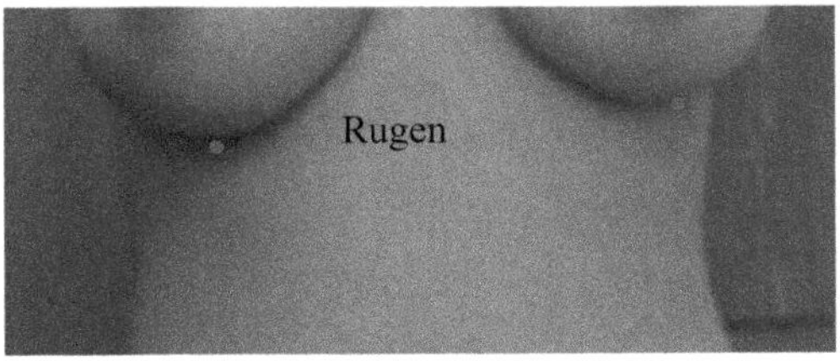

Fig. 2-148

Location

Let your partner sit and lie on the bed.

Technique

Press Rugen for 1 minute until your partner can feel some soreness and swelling.

❺ Push and rub Danzhong

Location

Danzhong is on the median line of the chest, at the midpoint of the line connecting the two nipples (Fig. 2-149).

Position

Let your partner sit or lie on the bed.

Technique

Push Danzhong upwards for 1 minute until your partner can feel numbness and swelling of the breast.

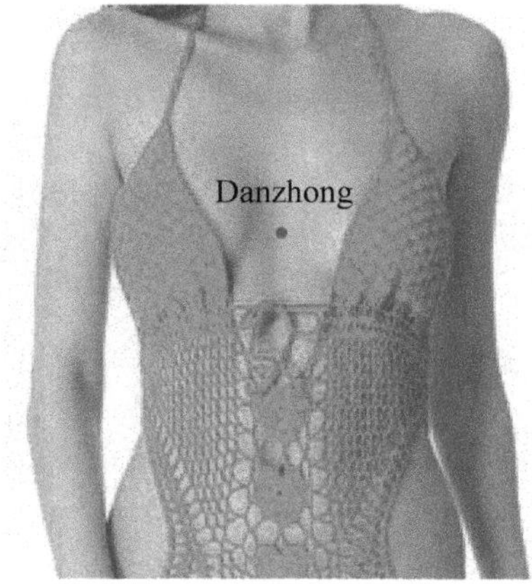

Fig. 2-149

❻ Pinch Shaoze

Location

Shaoze is next to the lateral corner of the little finger's nail (Fig. 2-150).

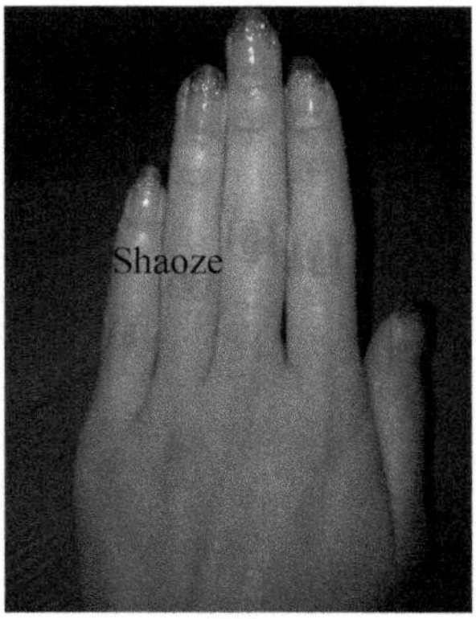

Fig. 2-150

Position

Let your partner sit or lie on the bed.

Technique

Pinch Shaoze for 20 sec with the finger nail and then let go, repeat 10 times.

❼ Press Zhongwan

Location

Zhongwan is on the median line of the upper abdomen, 13cm above the navel (Fig. 2-151).

Position

Let your Partner sit or lie on the bed.

Technique

Press Zhongwan with the thumb or middle finger for about 1 minute until your partner can feel some soreness and swelling.

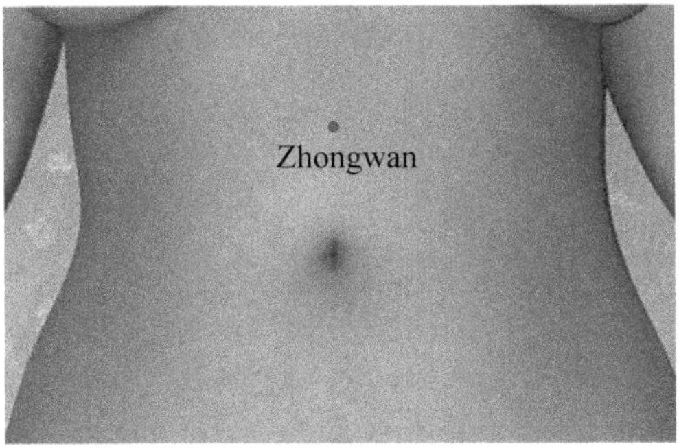

Fig. 2-151

❽ Rub Zusanli

Location

Zusanli is located at about 6.5 cm below the depression on the outer side of the knee, about one finger-width lateral to the crest of the tibia (Fig. 2-152).

Position

Let your partner lie on the bed.

Technique

Rub Zusanli for about 2 minutes until your partner can feel some soreness and swelling.

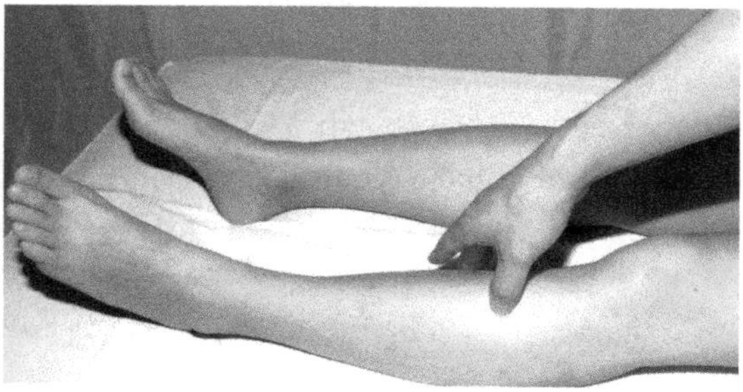

Fig. 2-152

❾ Press Taichong

Location

Taichong is located on the dorsum of the foot, in a depression distal to the junction of the first and second metatarsal bones (Fig. 2-153).

Position

Let your partner lie on the bed.

Technique

Press Taichong for half a minute.

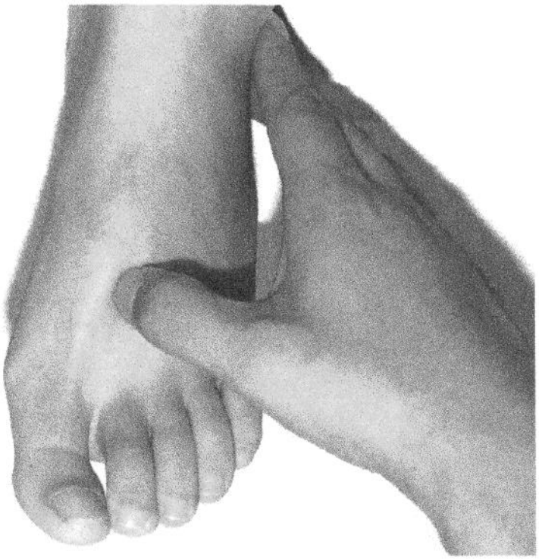

Fig. 2-153

Tips

1. Try to keep a happy mood during massage. Also, work on your nutrition; have more rib soup, chicken soup and fish soup to stimulate the milk secretion.

2. Please go and see a doctor if there are medical problems with the mammary glands.

Chapter Three

Forever Young -Beauty Massage

Get Rid of Facial Melasma and Freckles

There are a lot of factors for getting maculae, including the sun light, disease, medication, cosmetics, and emotions. People used to think it was normal to get maculae by their middle age, but they have become a common sight among young people as well. Although some people think that melasma and freckles are not a big deal, except for their influence on the looks, most girls would do anything to get rid of them.

According to Chinese medicine, melasma and freckles appear because of many reasons, such as obstruction of meridians leading to blood stasis and stagnation, so the blood cannot reach the face to nourish the skin. Metabolic waste products cannot be removed and the harmful substances wil remain inside the normal metabolic procedure leading to accumultaion which again shows in facial maculae. Sometimes they can be connected to diseases, such as ovarian cysts, fibroids, hyperplasia of mammary glandsand irregular menstruation. Therefore, be cautious when you see maculae.

Massage is a good alternative method to give treatment. It improves the facial skin quality. After a certain while of perseverance, the maculae on the face will fade.

Instructions

❶ Massage the sides of the face

Rub the face starting from the chin and lower jawbone to the back of the ear and then down to the shoulder, repeat 6 times. Then do the other side. This procedure can help to improve the blood circulation.

❷ Massage the mouth area

Rub from philtrum along nasolabial fold to Yingxiang next to the alar sidewalls and press it. Repeat 3 times until you can feel some heat.

❸ Massage the cheeks

Rub the cheeks in circles, on three layers from the outside of the face towards the inside. This does not only work on the skin but can also make the face slimmer.

❹ Rub the nose

Please rub the nose from nose tip to nose root. Then rub the corner of the nose and repeat 3 times.

❺ Wipe around the eyes

Please wipe from the inner corner to the outer corner of the eyes, repeat 6 times on both sides.

❻ Rub the forehead

Please write the Chinese character " 井 " in order to activate the collaterals.

❼ Press Xuehai

Xuehai is about 6.5 cm above the medial corner of the patella when the knee is flexed, on the bulge of the quadriceps muscle. Use appropriate strength to press the point for 3 minutes, until you can feel some soreness and swelling.

❽ Massage Ashi points

Directly massage the area of the maculae. Ashi points are local points of a disease; as the blood circulation is impeded, you can directly massage the area to break the stagnation (Fig. 3-1).

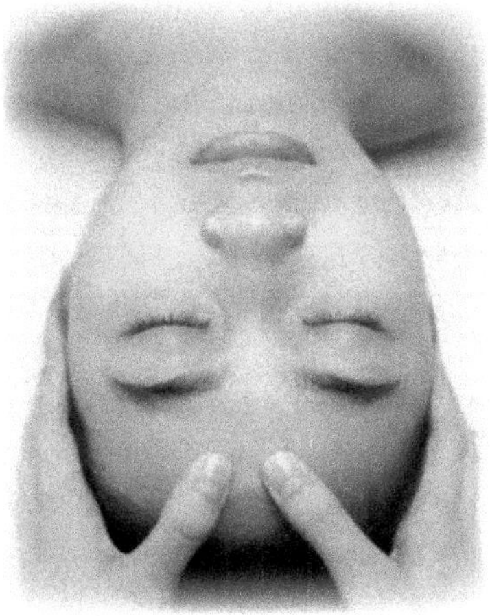

Fig. 3-1

Tips

1. Before the massage, clean the face thoroughly.
2. You can use a facial mask after the massage.
3. After the massage, you can pat the skin or press further acupoints on the face.

Fade off Stretch Marks

1. Stretch marks appear when the elastic fibres in the skin break because the skin is being over-stretched, causing atrophy. They may appear during the first six months of pregnancy and get more pronounced by the seventh month, as the baby then develops rapidly. So, irregular pink or purplish marks can show up on the belly. After giving birth, they can gradually recover and turn white, but they will not completely disappear.

2. According to Chinese medicine, stretch marks originate from innate deficiency and lack of skin nourishment.

3. Actually, if the mother-to-be takes care of her skin and her partner helps with massaging, stretch marks can be diminished or even eliminated.

4. Keep massaging the skin, especially the areas where

fat and marks appear easily, for example the breast, back, abdomen, bottom, the outer side of the leg and the knee. Massage can help to increase the elasticity and keep the blood circulation smooth, so the collagen fibers will not be torn and stretch marks will be prevented. Use appropriate strength so as not to harm the baby. Why not have a try?

Instructions

❶ Massage the breast

Have your partner seated. Warm and rub the breast with a hot towel and massage it with both hands covered entirely with olive oil until you can feel some heat. Then massage from the root of the breast to the area around the nipple. Please put a little amount of oil on the palm, and rub it between two hands till they turn warm. Then massage the breast in circles around the nipples starting from the cleavage to the outer edge.

❷ Massage the back

Please let your partner lie on the belly. Put a little amount of oil on the palm. Then massage the spine area from the middle line to the outside of the back, repeat 10 times.

❸ Massage the abdomen

Please let your partner lie on the bed. Put a little amount of oil on the palm. Then put your hands on both sides of the navel. Keep drawing circles in a clockwise direction, starting with small ones and getting bigger until they cover the whole abdomen.

❹ Massage the buttocks

Please let your partner lie on the bed. Put a little amount of oil onto the palms. Then put both of your hands under the buttocks and push upwards, then massage from inside out along the edges of the buttocks; do both sides.

❺ Massage the inner leg

Please let your partner lie on the bed. Put a little amount of oil on the palm. Then push from the knee to the hip and back again, repeat 10 times.

❻ Massage the knee

Please let your partner lie on the bed. Put a little amount of oil on the palm. Massage both knees in circles from the inside outwards (Fig. 3-2).

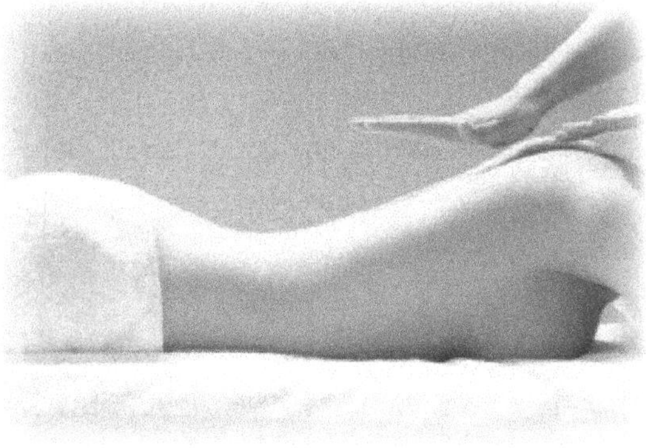

Fig. 3-2

Tips

1. For best results, keep massaging from the 3rd month of pregnancy to the 3rd month after giving birth.

2. It is best to use some massage oil, massage lotions, body lotions, infant oil, glycerin or lanolin oil.

3. During massage, please control your strength to avoid affecting the baby.

4. Please massage gently. If the strength is too much, the stretch marks will increase because the skin will be put under stress which can cause the collagen fibers to break.

Say Goodbye to the Dark Circles under Your Eyes

There are two factors of dark circles. One is vascular, it is due to poor blood circulation and dilation of blood vessels. People who suffer from allergic rhinitis or lack of sleep will get dark circles. The other factor is connected to pigmentation; accumulation of pigments (for example from bad quality make-up or rubbing the eyes) can lead to mild inflammation and pigmentary residuals.

According to Chinese medicine, the kidney commands the water and is reflected in the black colour. Kidney deficiency results in disturbances of the water metabolism. long term deficiency of kidney qi will result in disorders of blood and qi circulation. The eyes will lose nourishment, so dark circles appear under the eyes.

There are a lot of methods to get rid of the dark circles. The best method is massaging. The massage stimulates the blood circulation and accelerates the metabolism of waste products. The dark circles finally fade off.

Instructions

❶ Press above the eye socket

Let your partner sit on the chair. Please stand behind your partner and use the middle finger and the ring finger to press the upper ridge of the eye socket from the inner to the outer corner of the eyes. Please repeat this procedure 3 times to relax the skin muscle.

❷ Massage the eye corner

Please let your partner sit on the chair. Stand behind your partner and draw little circles with your ring finger from the inner to the outer corner of the eyes. Please repeat this procedure 5 times to help blood circulation.

❸ Press the lower corner of the eye

Have your partner seated. Stand behind her and use your ring fingers to massage the lower canthus in anti-clockwise circular movements. Repeat 5 times.

❹ Press Taiyang

Let your partner sit on the chair. Stand behind your partner and press Taiyang. Taiyang is located in a depression about one finger-width posterior to the lateral end of the eyebrow and the outer canthus. Press tightly, release for 3 seconds, then press from Taiyang back to canthus. Repeat 3 times.

❺ Press the lower canthus and Taiyang

Let your partner sit on the chair. Stand behind your partner and press the lower canthus, massage to Taiyang, using little circular movements. Repeat 5-10 times.

❻ Warm the eyes

Let your partner sit on the chair. Please stand behind your partner and rub your hands until they feel hot, then cover your partner's eyes (Fig. 3-3).

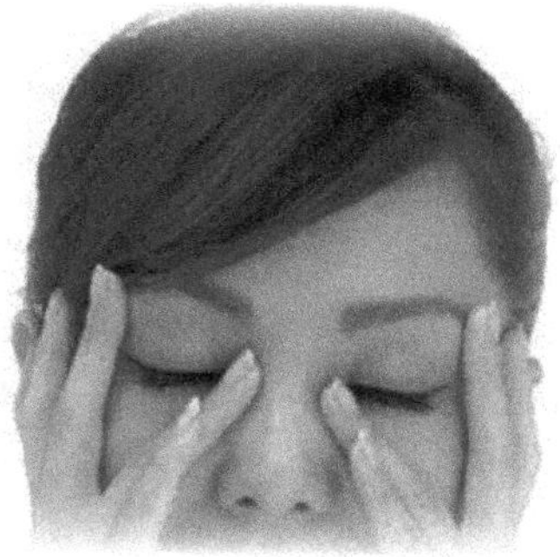

Fig. 3-3

Tips

1. Please stick to this sequence.
2. Please massage gently with eye cream to avoid wrinkles.
3. Keep massaging every day to avoid getting wrinkles.

Get Rid of Eye Pouches

Eye pouches are linked to genetic factors, age and living habits. Women usually start getting them in their thirties due to the fatty tissues, sometimes even due to edema. Since the lower eyelid is very thin, it will easily bulge out. Obviously, deficiency of sleep or poor blood circulation can also cause eye pouches.

According to Chinese medicine, eye pouches are mainly caused by a deficiency of kidney-yin. There is not enough essence to nourish the eyelids and there are problems with water metabolism, leading to kidney deficiency and edema manifesting in the lower eyelid.

Massage can get rid of eye pouches, except the ones brought about by genetic factors. Massage will stimulate the meridians and points around the eye area and activate the blood circulation around the eyes to remove the eye pouches. You will see positive results if you stick to it.

Instructions

❶ Press Jingming and Chengqi

Let your partner look upward and tap the inner eye corner (Jingming) 20 times with the ring finger. Jingming is located just next to the inner eye corner on both sides of the nose. The massage can activate the blood circulation. Chengqi is in a depression on the lower canthus, in a straight line under the pupil. This area is full of blood vessels, if the circulation is impeded, they will turn dark and dilate, forming eye pouches. Use your ringfinger to massage the point (Fig. 3-4).

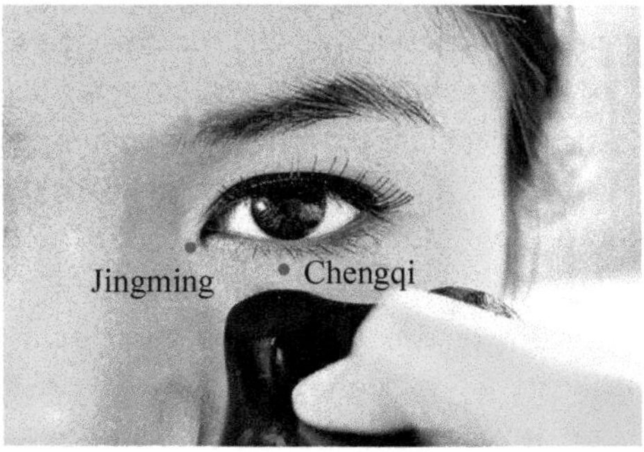

Fig. 3-4

❷ Press Taiyang

Pat from the inner eye corner to the outer corner and then gradually move to Taiyang and pull the skin 3 times. (Taiyang is in a depression on the temples) Massaging Taiyang can relieve the nerves of the brain and remove tiredness of the eyes.

❸ Massage the glabella

The position between the eyebrows is a place where a lot of active meridians pass. Parallel massage can comfort the nerves on the glabella. Please press the inner corner of the brow with the ring finger and press the outer corner with the middle finger. Rub the brow with the ring finger to the outer corner and push with both of the two fingers in the direction of the temple, repeat 3 times.

❹ Pull the eyelid

Moving the eyelid can improve and tighten the eye pouch. Put the forefinger and middle finger into a "V" shape and pull the skin from the inner corner to the outer corner right to the temple, repeat 3 times.

Tips

1. Clean the face before massaging, steaming will give you even better effects.

2. Use some eye cream for the massage to avoid friction of the skin.

3. Before massage, press points around the eyes, for example the corner and middle point of the brows (Yangbai and Sizhukong). Press hard and release gently , repeat 6 times.

4. Massage every day or every other day, 20 times are one course of treatment. This can prevent and eliminate dark circles as well as improving eye wrinkles if done in long term.

5. Follow the direction of muscles and massage perpendicularly to wrinkles.

Remove Eye Wrinkles

Eye wrinkles are so-called crow's feet, they appear between canthi and temples and they are symbols of aging. Eye wrinkles are caused endocrine hypo function decreased cellular activity of the fibre cells in the dermis, reduction of collagenous fibres and fraction, which all result in the decrease of skin elasticity. Besides, sunshine, dryness, coldness, hot water, facial expressions and smoking can also lead to the decrease of skin elasticity, thus resulting in the increase of eye wrinkles.

According to Chinese medicine, skin face is nourished by qi and blood, so lack or stagnation of qi and blood will cause wrinkles. Besides, irregular menstruation and other gynecological diseases caused by deficiency of the kidney, sleep disorders, poor diet, and increased vaginal discharge, frequent micturition, belly ache and lumbago caused by downward flow of damp heat can also lead to changes in the face and the increase of eye wrinkles.

Massage can make the eye skin tight and elastic; it is a very effective way to remove eye wrinkles.

Instructions

❶ Massage the skin on the sides of the eyes

Let your partner sit on a chair, stand behind your partner, apply some eye cream on the sides of the eyes and put your index and middle fingers onto the sides of the eyes and massage them slowly and softly and let your partner close his/her eyes. Pull your fingers backward to the ears, count from 1 to 5 and release your fingers. Repeat this 6 times.

❷ Massage the eyelids

Let your partner sit on a chair, stand behind your partner, apply some eye cream onto the canthus, cover it with cling film so it will penetrate quickly and remove it after 5 minutes. Massage the lower canthus with your index, middle and ring fingers from inside outwards, be gentle but firm and repeat 3 times. Put your thumb onto the eye socket between eyes and nose, massage the upper eyelid carefully with some pressure from the inside out and press Taiyang slightly harder with the middle and ring fingers. Keep the pressure for 5 seconds and release it for 3 seconds. Repeat once.

❸ Press the upper eye socket and eyebrow

Let your partner sit on a chair, stand behind your partner, press the upper eye socket and eyebrow slowly and lightly with your middle and ring fingers, move from the inside to the outside. Repeat 3 times.

❹ Massage the skin around the eyes

Let your partner sit on a chair, stand behind your partner, massage with ring fingers in small circular movements from the outer corner of the eye towards the eye socket in and then back to the outer corner. Repeat this 5 times to activate the skin around the eyes.

❺ Press the lower eyelid

Let your partner sit on a chair, stand behind your partner, and massage the lower eyelid in anti-clockwise circles from the eye socket towards the outer corner of the eye and Taiyang with your ring finger. Press slightly harder for 3 seconds and massage back to the eye socket. Repeat 3 times (Fig. 3-5).

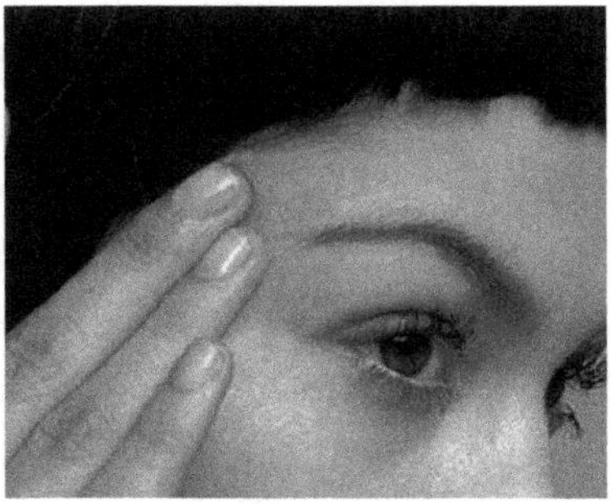

Fig. 3-5

Tips

1. Stick to the same sequence.

2. Too much eye cream will cause fat granules and too little will influence the effect.

Reduce Forehead Wrinkles

Forehead wrinkles can be seen when you lift your forehead and are a symbol of aging. Subcutaneous fat and water decrease with age, the dermis loses nourishment leading to a decrease of skin vitality, resulting in wrinkles. Facial expressions can also lead to wrinkles. Raising the eyebrows can weaken the recovering abilities of the forehead muscles and, in long term, lead to a decrease of elasticity of subcutaneous fibrous tissue. Raising the eyebrows squeezes the skin on the forehead and leaves lines which turn into wrinkles.

According to Chinese medicine, forehead wrinkles are due to a lack of blood or nourishment, stagnation of blood and blockage of channels.

Although wrinkles caused by aging cannot be prevented, massage can slow down the aging process of the skin and reduce wrinkles.

Instructions

❶ Massage the forehead

Let your partner sit on a chair, stand behind your partner and use your middle and ring fingers to massage Taiyang in circular movements.

❷ Massage the eyes

Let your partner sit on a chair, stand behind your partner, and massage from Taiyang down to the eyelid and around eye rim, repeat 5 to 6 times.

❸ Massage the nose

Let your partner sit on a chair, stand behind your partner, massage the nose from the upside downwards and rub the wings of the nose.

❹ Massage the cheek

Let your partner sit on a chair, stand behind your partner, carefully massage from the jaw to the ear, from the corner of the mouth to the ear and from the nose to the temple.

❺ Press Yangbai

Location

Yangbai is located on the forehead, right above the pupils and 3 cm from the superior border of the eyebrows.

Position

Let your partner lie on the bed

Technique

Sit behind your partner, massage Yangbai with both thumbs in a clockwise direction for 2 minutes and then in an anti-clockwise direction for 2 minutes. Try to provoke a feeling of distention spreading to the whole forehead.

❻ Press Yintang

Location

Yintang is located on the forehead, right in between the eyebrows.

Position

Let your partner lie on the bed.

Technique

Sit behind your partner, use both thumbs in turns to press from nasal root upward to Yintang, keep doing for two minutes until you provoke a feeling of distention in the forehead.

❼ Press Sizhukong

Location

Sizhukong is located above the outer canthus, in a depression at the end of the eyebrow.

Position

Let your partner lie on the bed.

Technique

Sit behind your partner, press Sizhukong with both thumbs in a clockwise direction for 2 minutes and then in an anti-clockwise direction for 2 minutes. Try to provoke a feeling of distention spreading to the whole forehead.

❽ Press Touwei

Location

Touwei is located above the temple, about 15 cm from the midline of the head and 1.5 cm above the hairline.

Position

Let your partner sit on a chair.

Technique

Sit behind your partner, massage Touwei with both thumbs in a clockwise direction for 2 minutes and then in an anti-clockwise direction for 2 minutes. Try to provoke a feeling of distention spreading to the whole forehead.

⑨ Press Tongziliao

Location

Tongziliao is located in a depression 1 cm from the outer canthus.

Position

Let your partner lie on the bed.

Technique

Sit behind your partner, press Tongziliao with thumbs and index fingers for half a minute, then massage in a clockwise direction for 1 minute and in an anti-clockwise direction for 1 minute (Fig. 3-6).

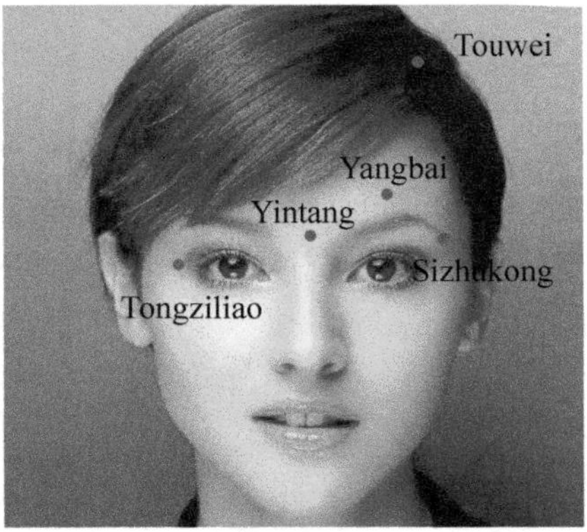

Fig. 3-6

⑩ Press Zusanli

Location

Zusanli is located at about 6.5 cm below the depression on the outer side of the knee, about one finger-width lateral to the crest of the tibia.

Position

Let your partner lie on the bed with knees bent slightly.

Technique

Sit behind your partner, massage Zusanli with both thumbs in a clockwise direction for 2 minutes and then in an anti-clockwise direction for 2 minutes (Fig. 3-7).

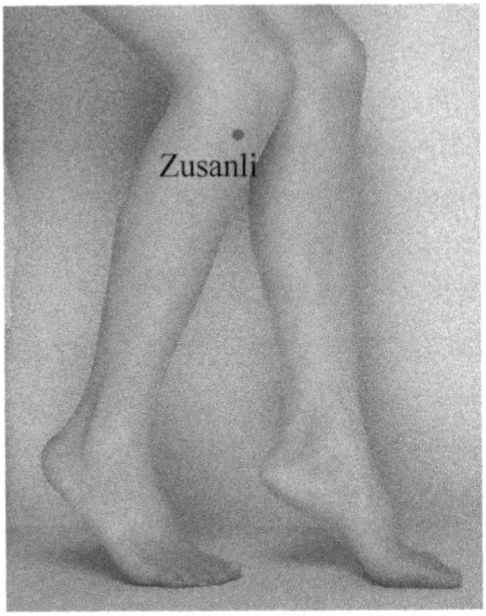

Fig. 3-7

Tips

1. Pay attention to the direction of the wrinkles when massaging. Wrong massage can increase the wrinkles.

2. Get half a grain of rice's eye cream with the third finger of the right hand, place it under the right eye and pull down the lower eyelid of the right eye with your left hand , watch out to do it very gently. The main goal is to smoothen the area and let the cream penetrate. Use the ring finger of the right hand to massage from the lower canthus of the right eye in clockwise movements extending to the whole eye. Massage until the cream is absorbed, repeat 4-5 times.

✿ Beautiful Breasts

Breasts are very important for the female beauty. The shape and size of breasts determine the beauty of breasts. Women's breasts start to mature at the age of 15 or 16, when the female curves are developing. Oversize and undersize development can influence the beauty of breasts.

Massage can promote the full development of breasts, increase the elasticity and skin quality, reduce superfluous fat, strengthen disease resistance of breasts and help the lobules of the mammary gland mature.

It is every woman's dream to have beautiful and healthy breasts, but not every woman is born with them. Apart from beauty products, there is an absolute safe and beneficial way – massage, which can have incredible effects. However, there needs to be some commitment to make a difference!

Instructions

❶ Massage breasts with palms

Let your partner lie on the bed, use the right palm to massage from the left collarbone to the breast root and back to the collarbone with soft and even strength, repeat 3 times. Do the same with your left hand on the right breast. Then use your right palm again to push from the sternum to the left breast and down to the armpit, repeat three times. Again, do the same thing with the left hand on the right breast. And do the same with left hand to right breast.

❷ Push the breasts

Let your partner lie on the bed, hold her right breast in your right hand and push it up slowly with comfortable pressure, release, and hold and push again, repeat 10-20 times. When pushing upward stop under the nipple. Do the same with your left hand on her left breast. Then pinch the nipples with the pads of your thumb and index fingers and pull them gently, repeat 10-20 times. If the nipples are inversed, you can repeat more or use more strength.

❸ Stroke the breasts

Let your partner lie on the bed gently, stroke her right breast with your left hand and her left breast with your right hand for 3 minutes. It doesn’t matter in which direction you stroke, but the three minutes of stroking are a very important part of the whole massage.

❹ Massage breasts with oil

Let your partner lie on bed, apply a thin layer of breast massage oil evenly on her breasts. Hold her right breast with your right hand, keep the fingers closed, do the same thing on the left side with the left hand. Use the right hand to push along the breast line while the left hand releases the breast at the same time. Repeat ten times and do the same thing on the other side.

❺ Use brush to massage breasts

Let your partner lie on bed, hold brushes in both and use them to massage the breasts in a circular motion around the nipples. Put hands on the lateral parts of the breasts, push them towards the sternum, use some pressure to brush to the armpit and then use some pressure to brush upwards. Now the shoulders should be rotating upwards. Gently brush back down to the sternum. Repeat ten times on both sides.

❻ Tapping and massaging the breasts

Let your partner lie on bed or sit on a chair, bend your middle or index finger to tap her breasts, starting gently and getting heavier, but watch out not to get too heavy. Start tapping the area under the nipple and tap the breasts in a circular motion leaving the nipples out, repeat 5 times (Fig. 3-8).

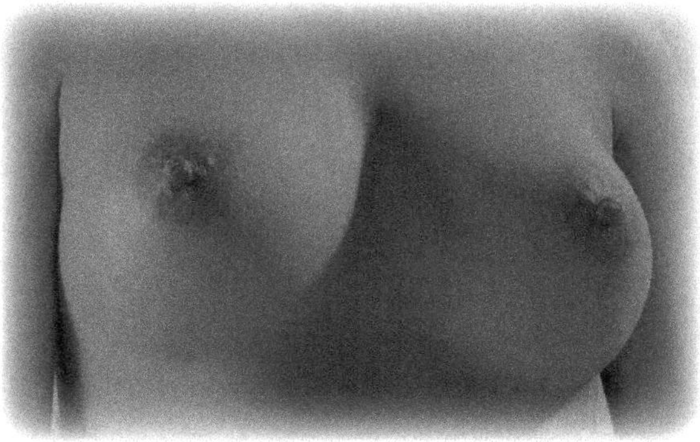

Fig. 3-8

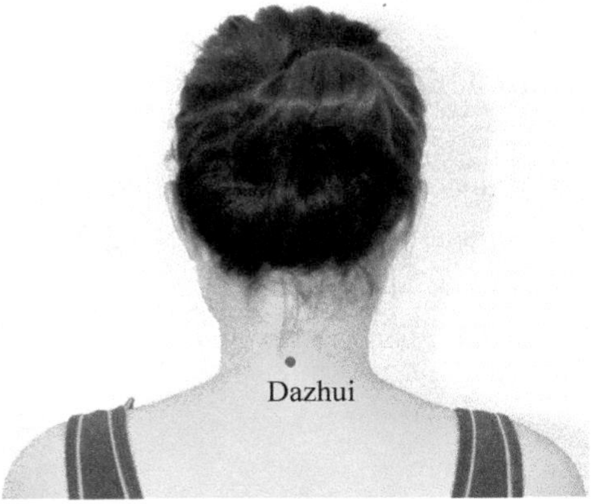

Fig. 3-9

❼ Press and rub Dazhui

Location

Dazhui is located on the lower neck, in a depression under the 7th cervical spine (Fig. 3-9).

Position

Let your partner lie on the bed or sit on a chair.

Technique

Let your partner lower his/her head slightly, press Dazhui with thumb or index finger for 1-2 minutes. There should be a feeling of distention when pressing.

❽ Press Guanyuan

Location

Guanyuan is located on the lower belly, right on the median line, about 10 cm under the umbilicus (Fig. 3-10).

Position

Let your partner lie on the bed.

Technique

Use the pads of index, middle and ring fingers to put pressure on Guanyuan and the area around it. Keep pressing for 15 minutes. Your partner should have an empty bladder, so it is best to do this after getting up or half an hour before going to bed.

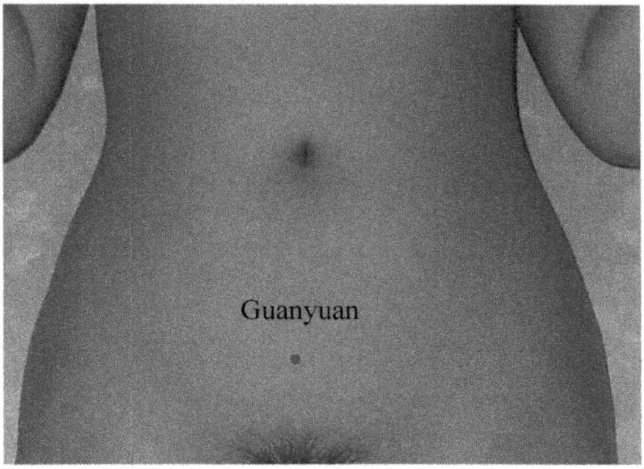

Fig. 3-10

Tips

1. The massage should be soft and gentle, don't use too much strength.

2. Use a nourishing cream to lubricate the breasts for massage.

✿ Eliminate Hip Fat

Women easily gain weight on the hips. Firstly, the gall-bladder meridian passes through the hip, so when it is affected by cold, fat can accumulate on the hips. Secondly, nowadays many people lack exercise and young people spend a lot of time sitting in front of their computers, which easily causes them to gain weight and have flaccid muscles. Thirdly, many people are fond of fried food and cold drinks, paying no attention to a healthy diet. They show with a lack of qi and blood which can also result in gaining weight.

Physical exercise can accelerate loosing weight and improve the strength of the hip muscles, but many people like patients with cardiovascular diseases cannot do large amounts of exercise. Thus, massage in the best option. Massage can not only get rid of excess fat and strengthen the hip muscles but also treat disease. Massage can make the belly and legs slimmer and raise your hip, so it can contribute to a slim figure.

Instructions

❶ Push the hip

Let your partner lie on the bed, put your hands onto the sides of your partner's buttocks, use strength to push towards the inside and let your partner contract the muscles of the buttocks 15 times. Use right and left hands alternatively to push your partner's buttocks and rub the skin with your palms until it is hot.

❷ Press hip in radial pattern

Let your partner lie on his/her stomach, overlap your palms, and push from the highest point of the hip downwards in a radial pattern. Repeat for 5 minutes.

❸ Push the sacrum

Let your partner lie on bed, push from sacrum downward to thigh, both hands alternatively, repeat 15 times. Rub Huantiao with fingers for 1 minute until there is a feeling of distention.

❹ Raise hip and twist waist

Let your partner lie on bed, hold his/her legs and let your partner raise the hip and twist the waist a few times.

❺ Push and pull the legs

Let your partner lie on the bed, use both hands to tightly hold one of your partner's knees, push and pull it 25 times and do the same on the other side (Fig. 3-11).

Tips

1. There will only be effects with long-term use of massage (at least 2 months) .

2. Do not force your partner or yourself to twist or raise the hip in case of possible backache.

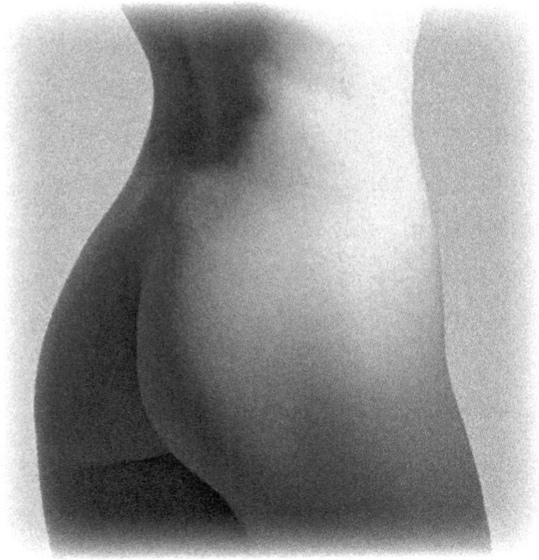

Fig. 3-11

Eliminate Belly Fat

Women also tend to gain weight on the belly. Exercise and massage are both good ways of losing weight. The popular belly massage for losing weight can be applied to many diseases related to the digestive system, nervous system and urogenital system as well as being a way to eliminate belly fat and strengthen the body.

Instructions

❶ Push and press belly in an ondular movement

Let your partner lie on the bed. Gently rub from the sides of the belly to the center, then change the direction. Put the left hand on top of the right hand with the fingers closed and place them on the belly. Push with the right palm and press back with the left palm, resulting in an ondular downward movement, just like waves in the water.

❷ Rub and squeeze both sides of the navel

Let your partner lie on the bed, slightly sqeeze the fatty tissue on both sides of the navel, then use a bit more strength to rub and squeeze until it becomes painful. This stimulates the fatty tissues.

❸ Kneading the belly

Let your partner lie on the bed, open your hands like dragon claws and knead the chubbiest part of the lower belly. Liver, gallbladder and spleen are in the upper part of the belly and the stomach is in the middle part. Rubbing these parts can help to get rid of fat. According to Chinese medicine, kneading is better than patting. If there is pain when kneading, the liver might not be functioning too well, so don't knead too hard. If there is pain on slight touch, you should go and see a doctor.

❹ Lift the belly

Let your partner lie on the bed, hold the chubbiest part of the belly with two hands and tell your partner to inhale deeply, lift the belly at the same time and then let your partner exhale and relax your grip.

Repeat 36 times.

❺ Massage belly in circles

Let your partner lie on the bed, put your hands on the belly with thumbs crossed and palms on the navel, tell your partner to inhale and tighten the belly, massage 36 circles in a clockwise direction, your hands and the belly will turn warm.

6. Pat the chubbiest part of the belly

Let your partner lie on the bed and pat the chubbiest part of the belly. Do it gently, just like patting on a baby's back after eating. Then form a hollow fist and pat the same area with it (Fig. 3-12).

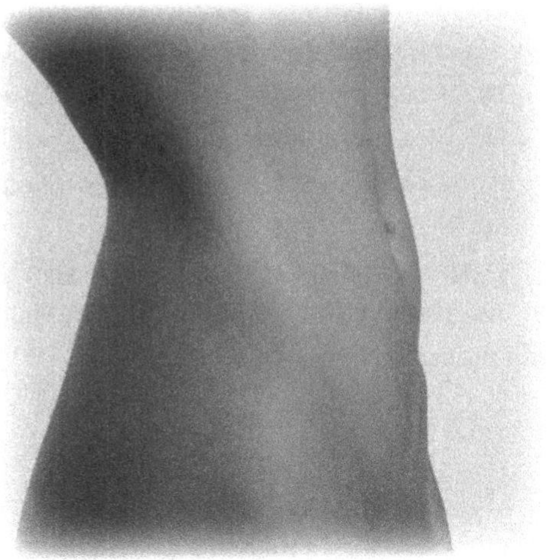

Fig. 3-12

Tips

1. As warming up, the part to be massaged should be rubbed in advance to relax the muscles before massage. Like this, the massage can be double efficient with half the effort.

2. Massage during a bath can have better effects. You can also massage during or after a shower if you want to quickly lose weight.

3. Each time, massage 3-5 minutes. No matter exercise or massage, the key to success is perseverance. It takes 2-3 weeks to see effects.

4. When massaging the belly, your partner should lie on the bed with the belt of the trousers loosened and only a thin layer of clothing on the belly. Sit on the left side of your partner. First push and press in an ondular downward movement starting from the upper belly, repeat 3-4 times, then use two fingers on top of each other to press Zhongwan, Tianshu and Guanyuan, 2-3 minutes each. Again, repeat the ondular movements 2-3 times. Massage once a day, don't do it on a full stomach or when your partner is hungry. People suffering from chronic diseases should take a few days' break after a month of massaging. Massaging once a day accompanied by a healthy diet will lead to losing weight.

5. You can also massage twice a day, once in the morning and once in the evening, each time 20-30 minutes. Make sure that you keep practicing every day.

Chapter Four

Intimate Comfort—
Partner Massage to Stimulate Sexual Desire

Stimulate Male Sexual Desire

Low sexual desire in men can show in a lack of sexual fantasies, a lack of desire in sexual activities, a lack of initiative or in a significant decline of sexual ability. In general, the sexual functions, impulses and ability start to get weaker in the forties, which is a normal physiological phenomenon. If the sexual function declines too quickly, it is advisable to go and see a doctor. If there are no organic or psychological causes, partner massage is a very good way to improve the sexual function.

Chinese medicine believes that a lack of sexual desire in men is due to factors such as kidney yin and yang deficiency, deficiency of blood, deficiency of vital energy and emotional stress.

Instructions

❶ Press Shangyang

Location

Shangyang is located at the radialis of distal segment finger, 4mm from the nail edge (Fig. 4-1).

Position

Let your partner lie on the bed.

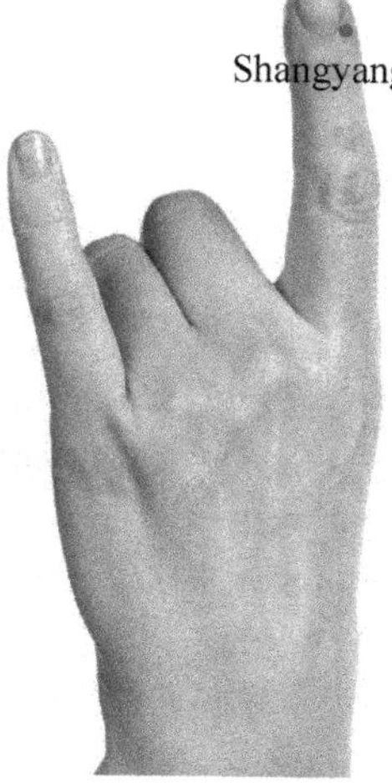

Fig. 4-1

Technique

Use index finger to massage Shangyang, for 10 minutes.

❷ Press Guanyuan

Location

Guanyuan is on the anterior midline, about 10 cm below the navel (Fig. 4-2).

Position

Let your partner lie on the bed.

Technique

Massage and stimulate Guanyuan using the finger pressing method, or use the left hand and right hand alternatively to massage

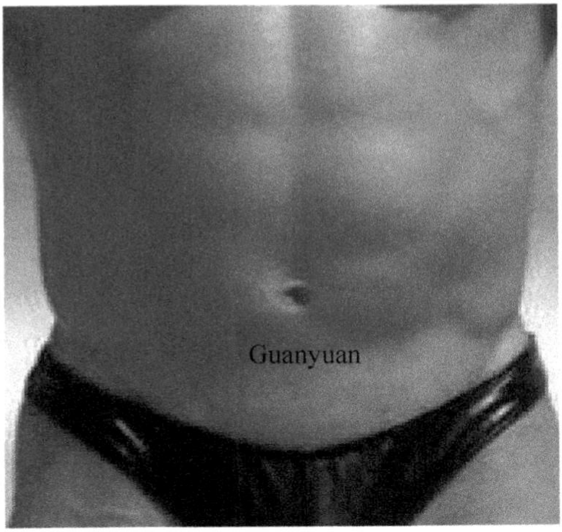

Fig. 4-2

the abdomen centering on the navel to stimulate the relevant acupoints on the conception vessel meridian.

❸ Stimulate the Sanyinjiao

Location

Sanyinjiao is one hand-width above the tip of the malleolus medialis behind the Tibia (Fig. 4-3).

Position

Let your partner lie on the bed.

Technique

Use yuur fingers to massage this acupoint.

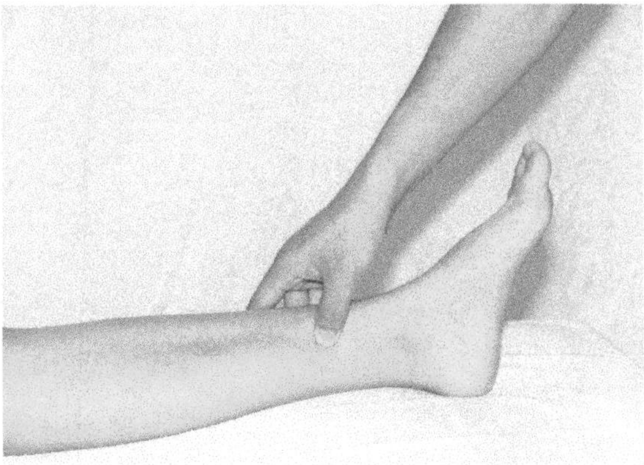

Fig. 4-3

❹ Stimulate Yongquan

Location

Yongquan is located on the bottom of the foot, in a depression in between the first third and the back two thirds of the sole of the foot (Fig. 4-4).

Position

Let your partner lie on the bed.

Technique

Take a hot footbath every night before going to sleep. Then, press Yongquan with your fingers or use a little stick to roll over the soles of your feet. Stimulation of this point can improve sexual ability.

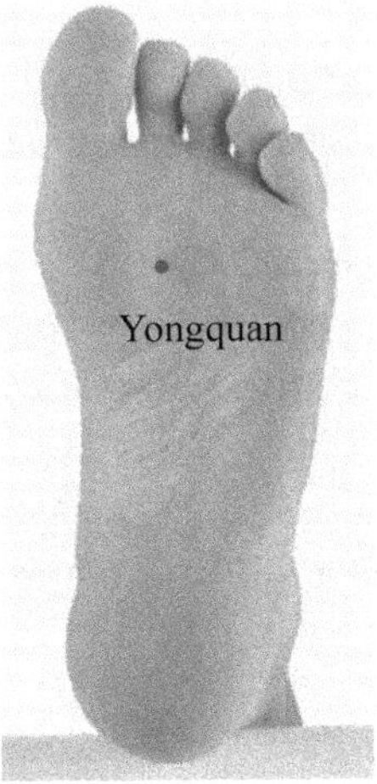

Fig. 4-4

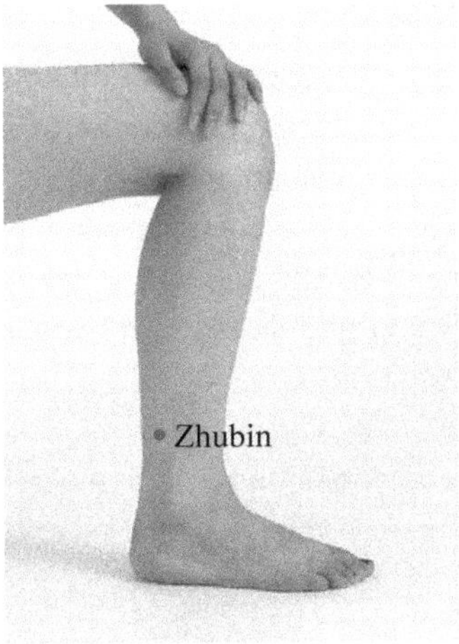

Fig. 4-5

❺ Stimulate Zhubin

Location

Zhubin is located at the inner side of the lower leg, about 6.5 cm above and behind Sanyinjiao (Fig. 4-5).

Position

Let your partner lie on the bed

Technique

Stimulating this acupoint can increase the sexual desire.

Tips

1. Prepare well for the massage, breathe into your belly and relax, try to give yourselves into it and be attentive to the details of excitement.

2. Use some massage oil or baby oil for lubrication.

3. The strength of massaging should be light at the beginning and slowly turn heavier until your partner can feel some soreness.

4. Your partner might feel aroused during the massage; don't be in a haste to make love, but rather rest for a little while before you have sex.

Relieve Sexual Strain

Sex is an instinctive and physical need of the human being. Normal sexual life is healthy and it can harmonize the relationship between husband and wife. However, excessive sexual activities can lead to sexual strain. The main symptoms for sexual strain are poor health, declining organ functions, premature aging reflecting in soreness and weakness of waist and knees and low spirits.

TCM believes that excessive sexual activities will consume kidney qi, cause sterility and premature aging, weaken the body's self-defence leading to inefficiency in work and learning or even do damage to the body.

Instructions

❶ Press and rub Mingmen

Location

Mingmen is located below the spinous process of the second lumbar vertebra (Fig. 4-6).

Position

Let your partner lie on the bed.

Technique

Use the thumb to press and rub Mingmen first in a clockwise and

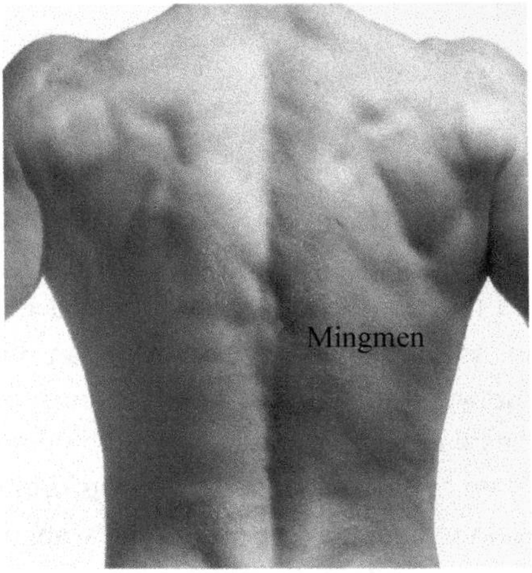

Fig. 4-6

then in an anti-clockwise direction until it feels sore and distended.

❷ Press and rub Guanyuan

Location

Guanyuan is located on the anterior midline, about 10 cm below the navel (Fig. 4-7).

Position

Let your partner lie on the bed.

Technique

Stand to the side of your partner. Use the thumb to press and rub Guanyuan first in a clockwise and then in an anti-clockwise direction,

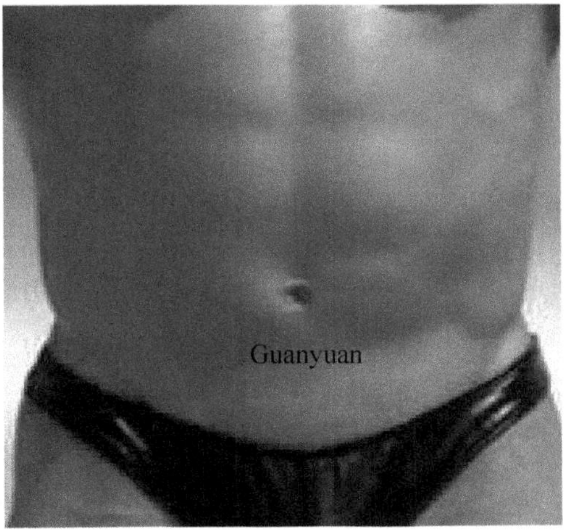

Fig. 4-7

2 minutes each, until it feels sore and distended.

❸ Press and rub Qihai

Location

Qihai is located on the anterior midline, about 5 cm below the navel (Fig. 4-8).

Position

Let your partner lie on the bed.

Technique

Use the thumb or middle finger to press and rub Qihai first in a clockwise and then in an anti-clockwise direction, 2 minutes each. Alternatively, you can also use a moxa stick on Qihai until it feels

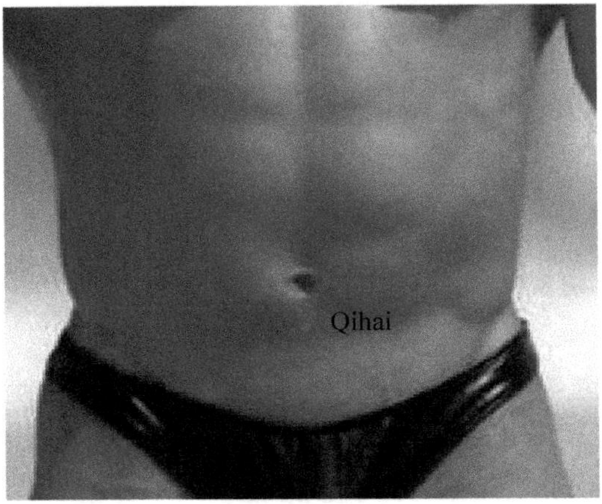

Fig. 4-8

warm and the skin turns red.

❹ Press and rub Shenshu

Location

Shenshu is located on the lower back, about 5 cm lateral to the lower border of the spinous process of the second lumbar vertebra (Fig. 4-9).

Position

Let your partner lie on the bed.

Technique

Use both thumbs to press Shenshu for half a minute, then press and rub Shenshu first in a clockwise and then in an anti-clockwise

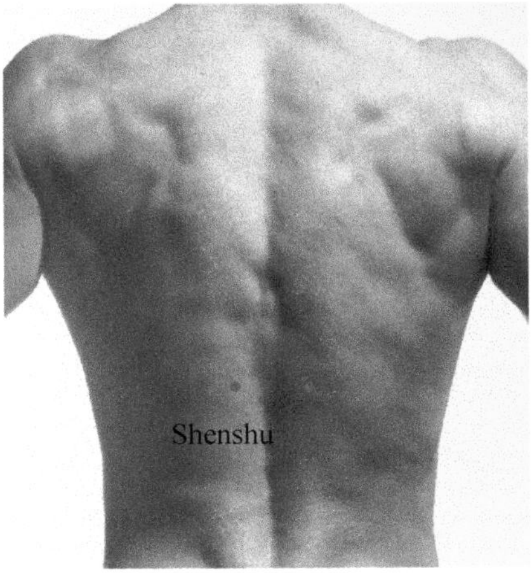

Fig. 4-9

direction, 2 minutes each, until it feels sore and distended.

❺ Press and rub Taixi

Location

Taixi is located in the depression between the tip of the medial malleolus and the Achilles tendon (Fig. 4-10).

Position

Let your partner lie on the bed.

Technique

Hold your partner's ankle. Use the thumb pad to press and rub Taixi first in a clockwise and then in an anti-clockwise direction, 2 minutes each, until it feels sore and distended.

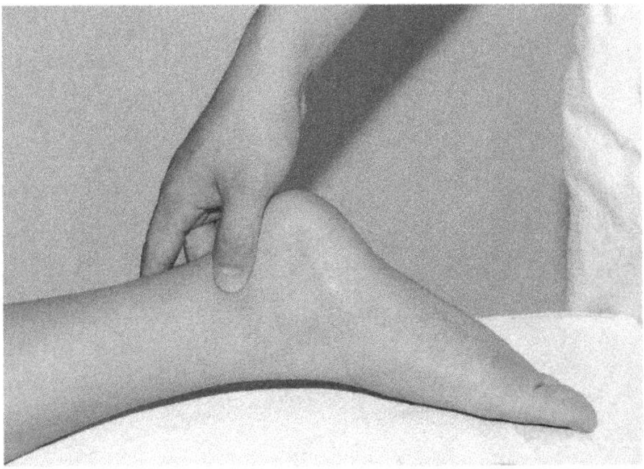

Fig. 4-10

6. Press Huiyin

Location

Huiyin is located in the middle of the perineum (Fig. 4-11).

Position

Let your partner lie on the bed.

Technique

Your partner lies on the back with the thighs slightly opened. Use your middle finger to press Huiyin in a clockwise and an anti-clockwise direction, 2 minutes each.

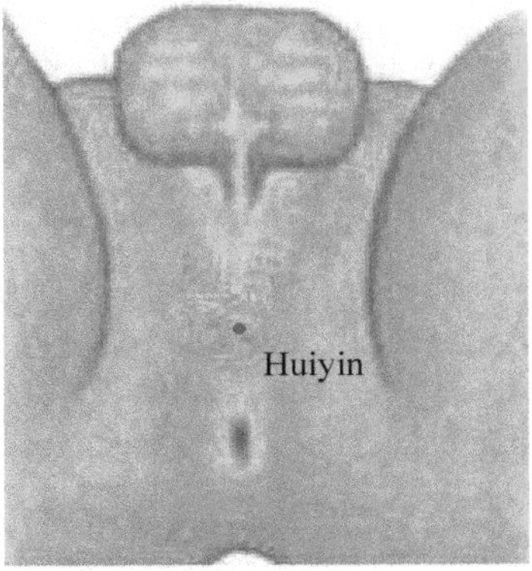

Fig. 4-11

Tips

1. Massage once a day, your partner should feel relaxed. Be gentle, don't let your partner feel pain.

2. It will take some time to see the effects of this massage, be patient and try to stick to it.

3. There will only be good results if your partner can find a balance between exertion and relaxation. Doing more physical exercises can help.

Stimulate Female Interest in Sexuality

If a woman loses interest in sexuality, it may show in many ways, such as fear, disgust, physical resistance, reluctancy, lack of participation, no response to caressing, lack of pleasure, no or little sexual secretions, tightening up, vaginal soreness during sex or the inability to have an orgasm. Reasons leading to loss of sexual interest include overwork, problems of the nerve system, suppression of sexual desire, over-indulgence in sexual pleasure, having sex at an early age, fear of pregnancy, coitus interruptus before the orgasm, etc. Also, side-effects of drugs or chronic diseases may lead to a disinterest in sex.

Chinese medicine believes that disinterest in sexuality is caused by inherent or postnatal deficiencies, emotional injuries, weakness due to diseases or abundant phlegm-damp.

Instructions

❶ Press Jiaosun

Location

Jiaosun is located right above the highest point of the ear (Fig. 4-12).

Position

Let your partner lie on the bed.

Technique

Insert your finger into the auditory meatus of your partner, and press it a little hard.

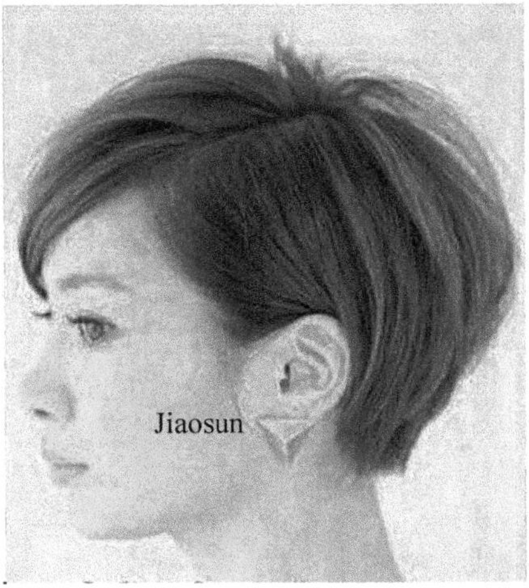

Fig. 4-12

❷ Press Zhongfu

Location

Zhongfu is located lateral to the first intercostal space (Fig. 4-13).

Position

Let your partner lie on the bed.

Technique

Use your thumb to slowly massage from the base of the neck to the clavicula.

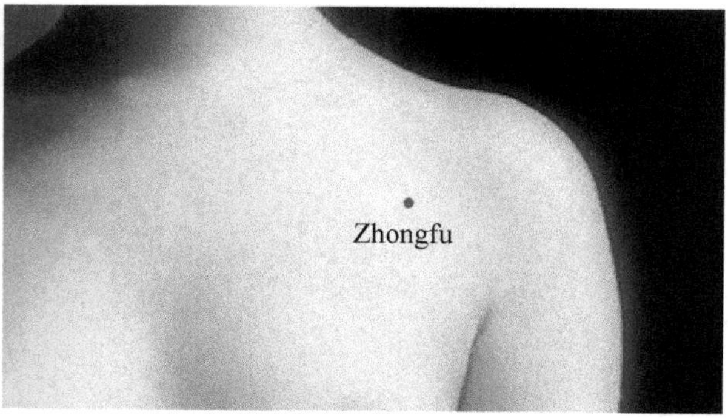

Fig. 4-13

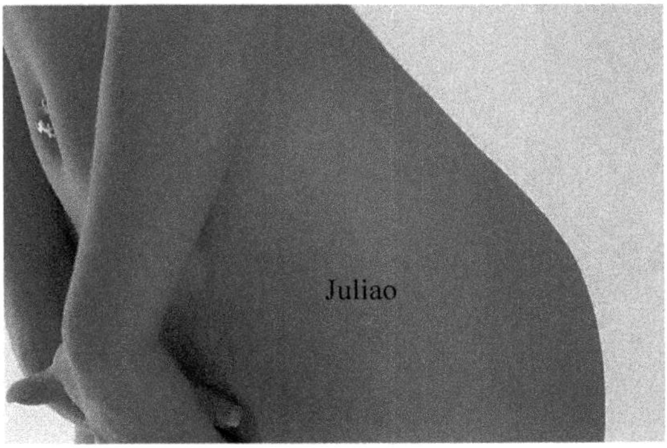

Fig. 4-14

❸ Press Juliao

Location

Juliao is located midway between the protuberance of the iliac spine and the greater trochanter (Fig. 4-14).

Position

Let your partner lie on the bed.

Technique

Gently press from the hipbone to the symphysis, pay attention not to use too much strength.

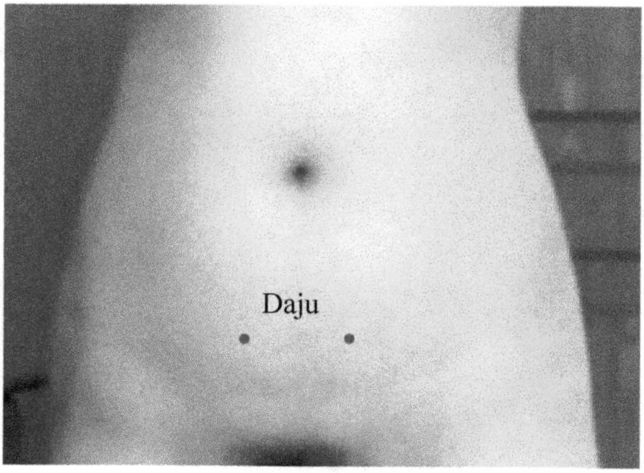

Fig. 4-15

❹ Massage Daju

Location

Daju is located on the lower abdomen, about 6.5 cm lateral to the midline and two "cun" below the navel. "cun" refers to a measurement unit, the distance between the navel and the pubic bone is 5 "cun" (Fig. 4-15).

Position

Let your partner lie on the bed.

Technique

Adjust the pressure to your partner's reaction. The goal of pressing this point is to promote the blood circulation and thus arouse your partner.

❺ Press Tianzhu

Location

Tianzhu is located on the lateral border of the trapezius muscle, above the transverse process of the second cervical vertebra, about 2 cm from the midline (Fig. 4-16).

Position

Let your partner lie on the bed.

Technique

Gently rub Tianzhu with your thumbs, this point is believed to have the effect of foreplay. This acupoint is the most effective one for women who sit in the office all day long.

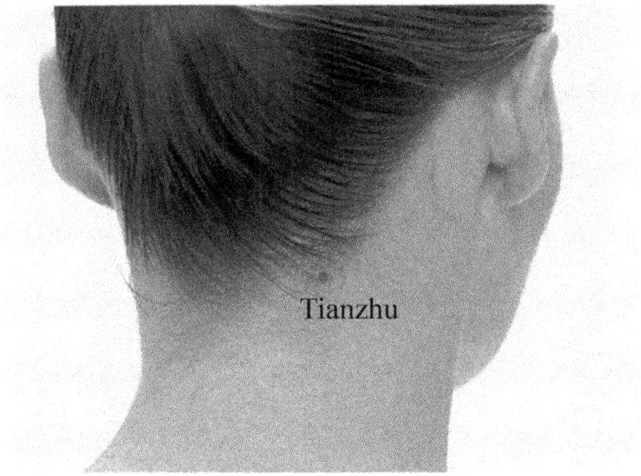

Fig. 4-16

❻ Press the Danzhong

Location

Danzhong is on the median line, right in between the nipples (Fig. 4-17).

Position

Let your partner lie on the bed.

Technique

Push Danzhong until your partner frowns slightly.

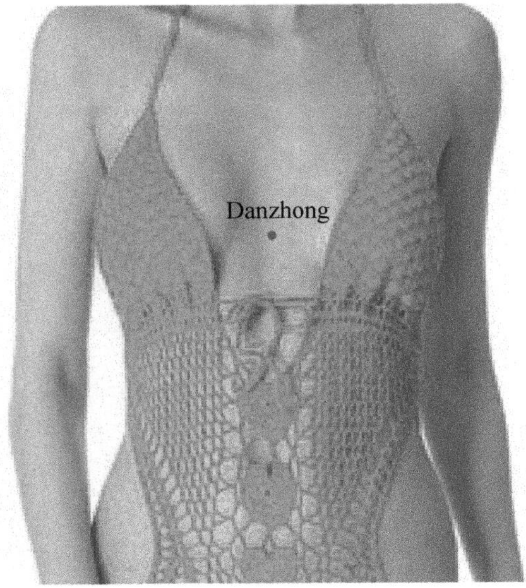

Fig. 4-17

❼ Press Yongquan

Location

Yongquan is located on the bottom of the foot, in a depression in between the first third and the back two thirds of the sole of the foot (Fig. 4-18).

Position

Let your partner lie on the bed.

Technique

Usually Yongquan is massaged with heavy pressure, but for arousal it is rather massaged lightly. There is an important nerve passing through Yongquan which can sexually stimulate a woman.

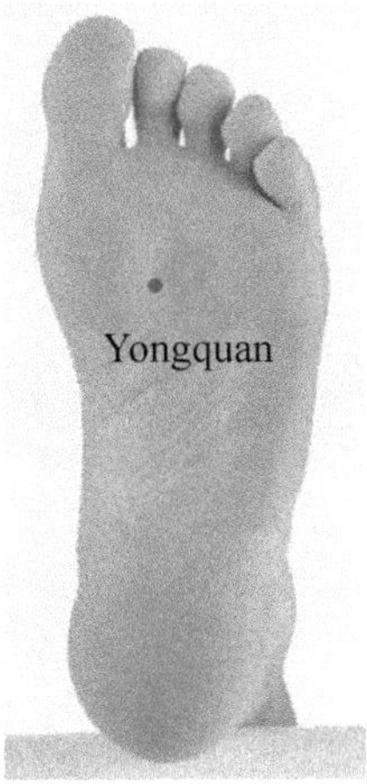

Fig. 4-18

❽ Press Dadun

Location

Dadun is next to the posterior corner of the nail on the lateral side of the big toe (Fig. 4-19).

Position

Let your partner lie on the bed.

Technique

Use your finger to apply pressure on Dadun.

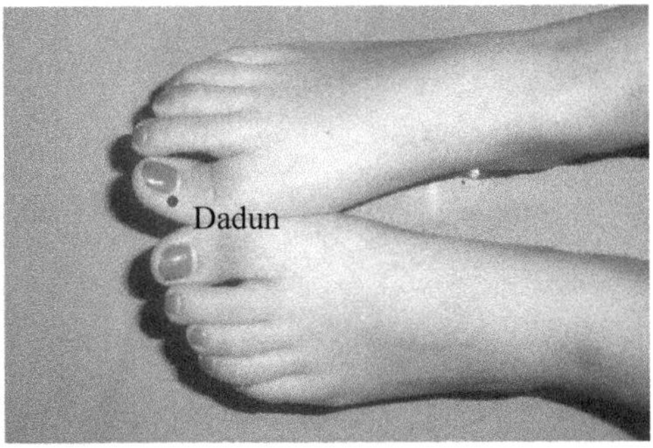

Fig. 4-19

❾ Press Weizhong

Location

Weizhong is located in the center of the popliteal crease (Fig. 4-20).

Position

Let your partner lie on the bed.

Technique

Gently press Weizhong with your finger can also enhance sexual excitement of your partner.

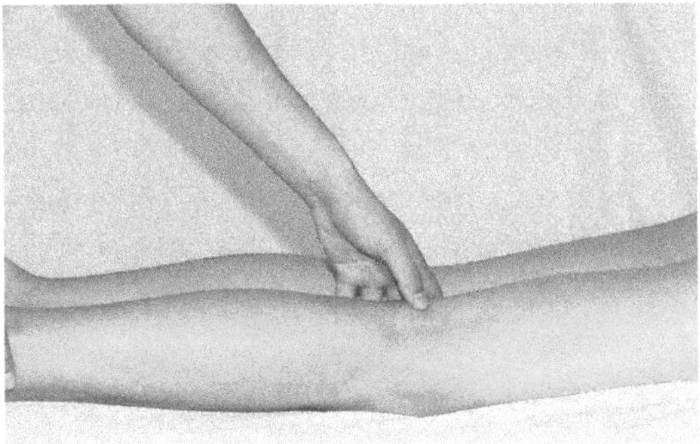

Fig. 4-20

Tips

Any of the mentioned techniques can also be applied by itself. Don't be too ambitious, but rather keep doing the massage for one or two months, then you will certainly see results.

Strengthening the Erection

Erectile dysfunction is a common male disease, meaning that the erection is insufficient to have or finish sexual intercourse, leaving the partner helpless or bitter. The reasons include organic causes such as excessive masturbation and prostatitis; systemic diseases such as hypertension or diabetes; and mental factors such as low confidence and worries about failure.

The Chinese medicine believes that ED is caused by deficiency of qi and blood, deficiency of liver and kidney, malnutrition of the urogenital region that are caused by an overindulgent sexual life, exhaustion of brain and physical strength, emotional disorder, irregular diet and so on.

Instructions

❶ Massage Yongquan

Location

Yongquan is located on the bottom of the foot, in a depression in between the first third and the back two thirds of the sole of the foot (Fig. 4-21).

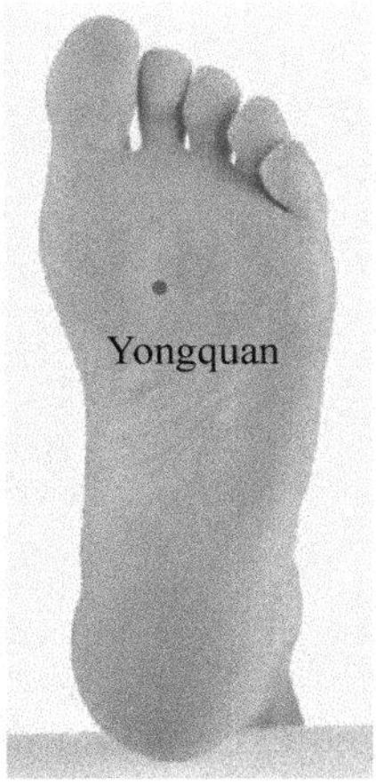

Fig. 4-21

Position

Let your partner lie on the bed

Technique

Use left hand to massage Yongquan on the right foot and the right hand to massage it on the left foot, 100 times each. You get the best effects after a hot footbath in the evening.

❷ Press and rub Qihai, Shenque, etc.

Location

Shenque is the center of navel; Qihai is on the anterior midline of the lower abdomen, about 5 cm below the navel (Fig. 4-22).

Position

Let your partner lie on the bed

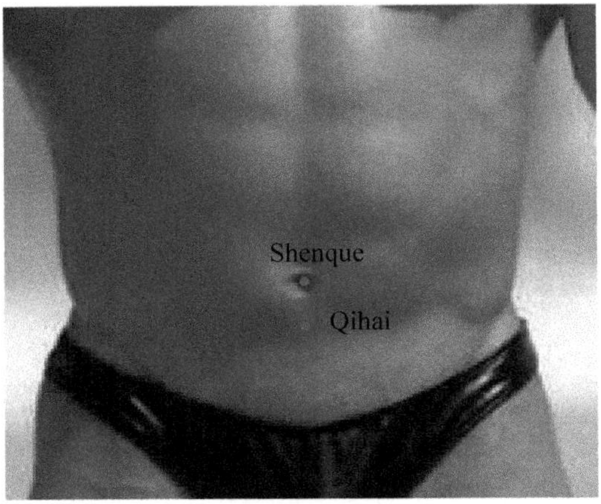

Fig. 4-22

Technique

First use the root of the palm to press Shenque with gentle and deep strength for about 5 minutes until your partner feels warm under the navel. Then use thenar to press and rub Qihai, Guanyuan, and Zhongji for about 2 minutes each. To finish off, rub Guanyuan, Qihai with palm for about 3 minutes until your partner feels warm in the lower abdomen.

❸ Press and rub Shenshu, Mingmen, etc.

Location

Shenshu is located on the lower back, about 5 cm lateral to the lower border of the spinous process of the second lumbar vertebra. Mingmen is on the posterior midline, under the spinal process of the second lumbar vertebra (Fig. 4-23).

Position

Let your partner lie on the bed.

Technique

First use light pressure to press and rub Shenshu and Mingmen for 2 minutes each, until your partner gets a feeling of soreness and distention. Then massage Ciliao and Zhongliao with your thumb for about six minutes each and with more pressure for one minute each. Finally, press and rub Yaoyangguan until your partner gets a warm feeling in the lower abdomen.

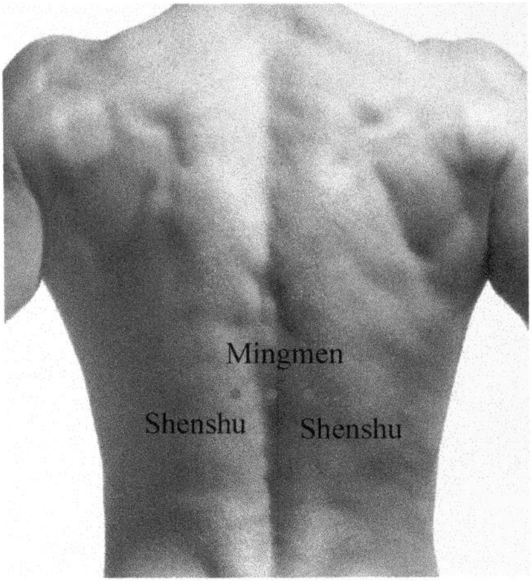

Fig. 4-23

❹ Press and rub Xinyu, Guanyuan, etc.

Location

Xinshu is located on the back, about 5 cm lateral to the spinous process of the fifth thoracic vertebra, Guanyuan is on the anterior midline, about 10 cm below the navel (Fig. 4-24, 4-25).

Position

Let your partner lie on the bed

Technique

Massage the Xinshu, Zhongwan, Guanyuan, Qihai and Zusanli for 1 minute each. Rub and press Xinshu and Zhongwan to strenghten the source of qi and blood. Guanyuan and Qihai strengthen the lower energizer and Zusanli harmonizes the ying and wei qi, invigorates the stomach and spleen and replenishes qi.

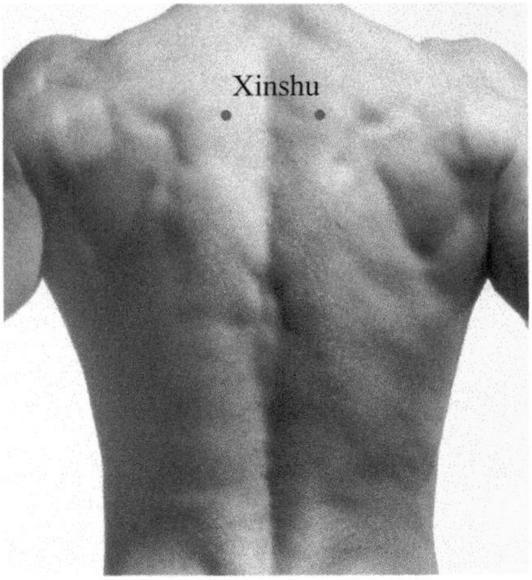

Fig. 4-24

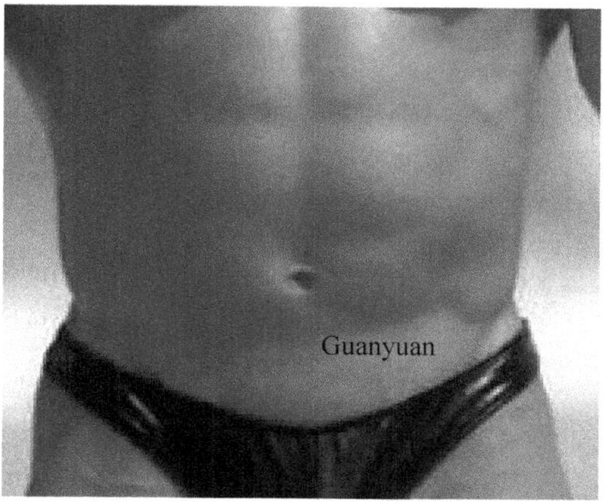

Fig. 4-25

Tips

1. When massaging, don't overdo it or be impatient. If it is done long-term, the effects will be much better.

2. For massage, the skin of the pubic area should be clean and healthy, don't massage on skin lesions or if there is inflammation. Gently massage once a day, try to relax, as the effects will be much better if you relax. The massage should not be painful.

3. After using the mentioned techniques for two to three weeks, erection may happen during massage. If it is not hard enough, then the penis and testes can be gently pulled. If the erection is hard enough, then just gently pull the testes. The

husband can first do this by himself, after about three weeks, the wife can take over, gradually starting to have sexual intercourse. This method works very well for functional ED; for ED due to organic causes, it should be combined with other therapeutic measurements.

Prolong Male Sexual Performance

Premature ejaculation is a common problem in males, meaning that the ejaculation happens too quickly, making it difficult to satisfy the partner. There are many psychological factors contributing to it, such as worrying about failure, long-term masturbation, lack of sexual knowledge, an unharmoniuos relationship, long-term inhibition, or the wife requesting to finish intercourse. Diseases such as urethritis, prostatitis, cytospermitis, benign prostatic hyperplasia, diabetes or cardiovasclar diseases can all contribute to premature ejaculation.

Chinese medicine believes that the occurrence of premature ejaculation is caused by many factors. For example, deficiency (deficiency of kidney, heart, and spleen) and damp-heat of liver and gallbladder are important factors. Inherent deficiency or masturbation, excessive sexual life, kidney deficiency impairing the storage of sperms, spermatorrhea, and mental and physical exhaustion can all cause premature ejaculation.

Massage has its own advantages in the prevention and treatment of premature ejaculation; it is simple and has no side-effets, making it a healthy way of home health care.

Instructions

❶ Press Sanyinjiao on both sides

Location

Sanyinjiao is located on the medial side of the calf, a hand-width above the tip of the inner ankle bone (Fig. 4-26).

Position

Let your partner lie on the bed.

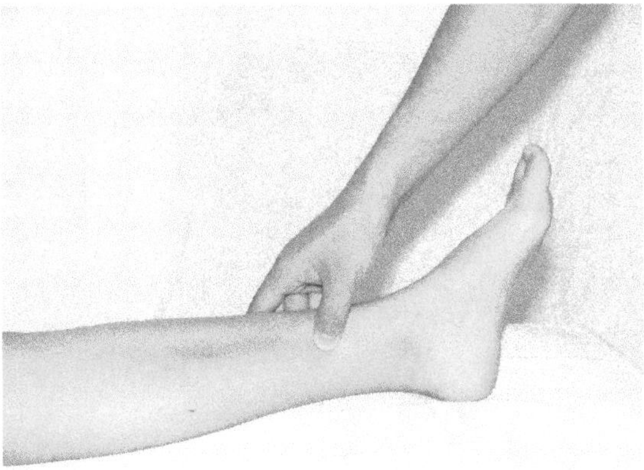

Fig. 4-26

Technique

Press Sanyinjiao on both sides alternatively, contract the lower abdomen and pull the anus up and relax again. Keep doing this for 30-40 minutes once or twice a day.

❷ Press on Shangxing and Baihui.

Location

Shangxing is on the midline of the head, about 3.5 cm behind the frontal hairline (Fig. 4-27). Baihui is on the intersection of the axis of the two ears with the midline of the head (Fig. 4-28).

Position

Let your partner sit on the bed or chair.

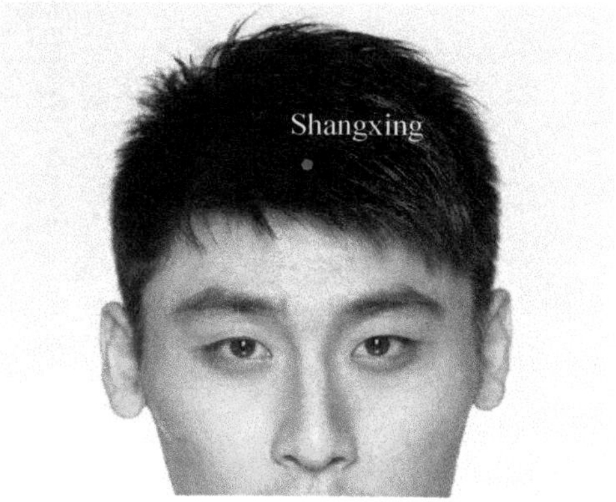

Fig. 4-27

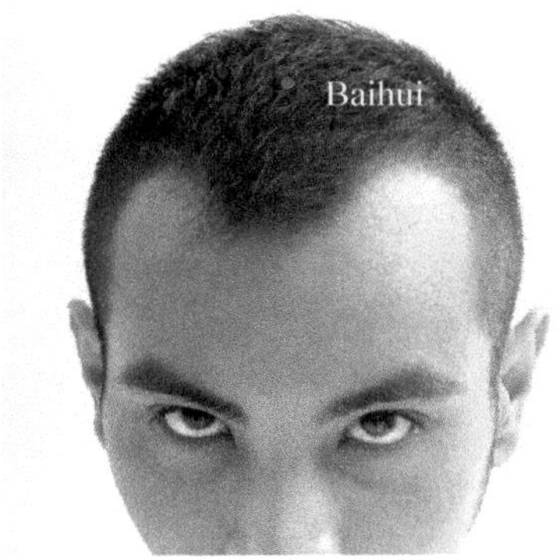

Fig. 4-28

Technique

Let your partner keep his eyes closed and relax. The points to use are Shangxing, Baihui, Tongtian, Jianjing, Zhongfu, Shenmen, Laogong, and other points on the head. Use tapping, pressing, rubbing, etc. techniques to massage for 30-40 minutes.

❸ Press on Zhongwan and Qihai

Location

Zhongwan is on the anterior midline, about 13 cm above the navel. Qihai is on the anterior midline, about 5 cm below the navel (Fig. 4-29).

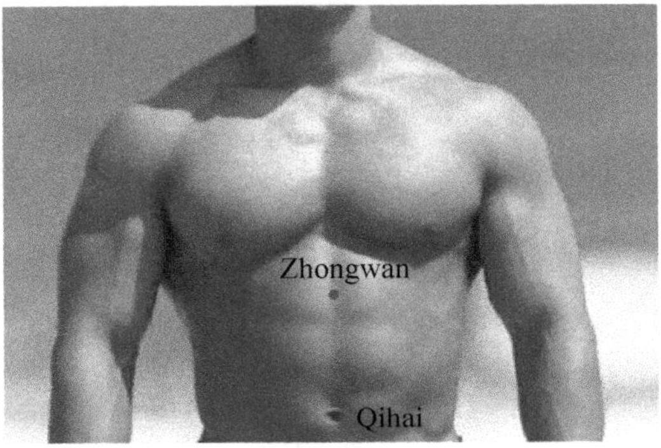

Fig. 4-29

Position

Let your partner lie on the bed.

Technique

Let your partner keep his eyes closed and relax. The points used are Zhongwan, Qihai, Guanyuan, Zhongji, Tianshu, Zusanli, Sanyinjiao, and Laogong. Use techniques like pressing, rubbing, tapping, etc., for about 30-40 minutes a day, 5 times a week, and keep doing it for one month.

❹ Massage Xinshu and Mingmen

Location

Xinshu is located below the spinal process of the fifth thoracic vertebra, about 5 cm lateral to the posterior midline. Mingmen is located on the midline, under the spinal process of the second lumbar vertebra (Fig. 4-30).

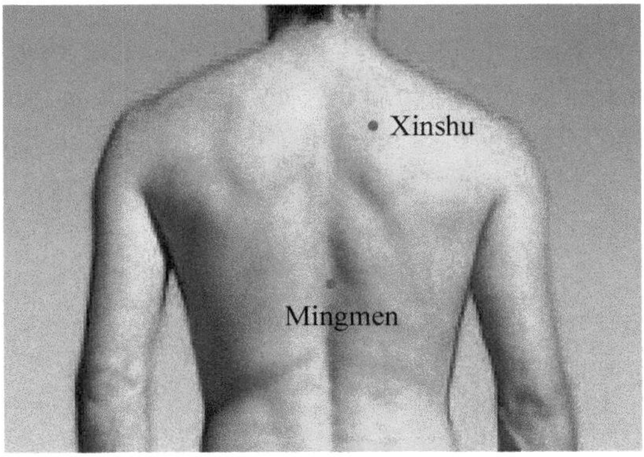

Fig. 4-30

Position

Let your partner lie on the bed.

Technique

Let your partner keep his eyes closed and relax. The points pressed are Xinshu, Ganshu, Shenshu, Mingmen, Yangguan, Huantiao, Kunlun, and Weizhong .Use techniques like pressing, rubbing, tapping, etc., for about 30-40 minutes a day, 5 times a week, and keep doing it for one month.

Tips

1. Your hand should be soft and gentle, avoid harsh movements as well as superfluous movements of the waist and legs.
2. The mentioned techniques should be applied long-term, avoid being impatient.

Eliminating Vaginal Spasm

Vaginal spasm is an involuntary contraction of the muscles of the opening and the outer third of the vagina, making it difficult to have sexual intercourse. It can occur to women of any age. It can be caused by many reasons, such as disorders of the uterus, vagina, anus and abdomen. Most of it is due to mental reasons though, like an unhappy marriage, problems with the husband, fear of sexual intercourse or stress. If the first sexual experience was linked to pain or violence, women will often relate sexual intercourse to pain and tighten up.

Chinese medicine believes that vaginal spasms are mostly caused by internal injuries. Emotional imbalance, rage affecting the liver, stagnation of liver qi or deficiency of kidney yin can all lead to vaginal spasms when having sex. The key to eliminating the spasms lies in understanding the causes. If they are caused by organic diseases, they will disappear when the lesions are cured. If they are caused by psychological obstacles, psychological counseling should be given first, but massage will help the treatment.

Instructions

❶ Press Guanyuan

Location

Guanyuan is located on the anterior midline, about 10 cm below the navel (Fig. 4-31).

Position

Let your partner lie on the bed.

Technique

Press Guanyuan with your thumb for about one minute until your partner can feel some soreness and distention.

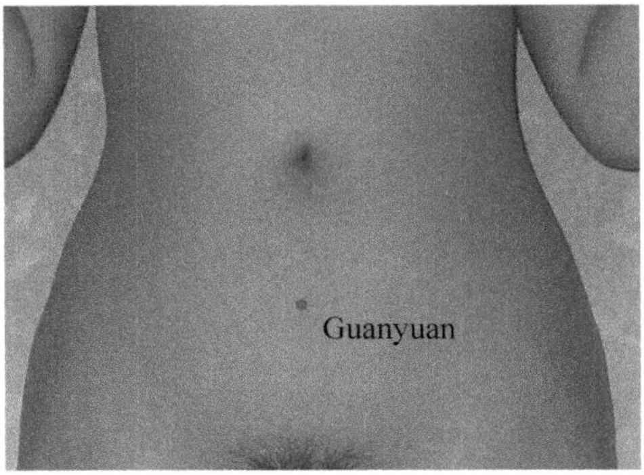

Fig. 4-31

❷ Press Qugu

Location

Qugu is on the anterior midline, right above the symphysis (Fig. 4-32).

Position

Let your partner lie on the bed.

Technique

Press Qugu with your thumb for about two minutes and massage in a clockwise direction for another two minutes until your partner can feel some soreness and distention.

❸ Press Huiyin

Location

Huiyin is in the middle of the perineum (Fig. 4-33).

Position

Let your partner lie on the bed.

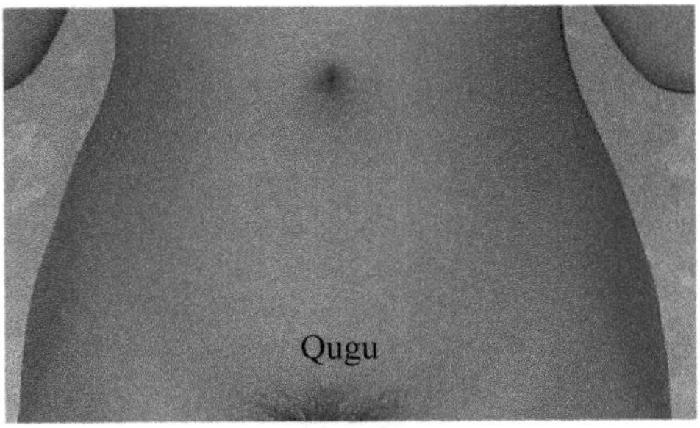

Fig. 4-32

Technique

Keep the thighs slightly open and press Huiyin in a clockwise and in an anti-clockwise direction for about two minutes.

Tips

1. Try to relax and massage gently.
2. For a significant improvement, keep doing for 1-2 months, don't be impatient.

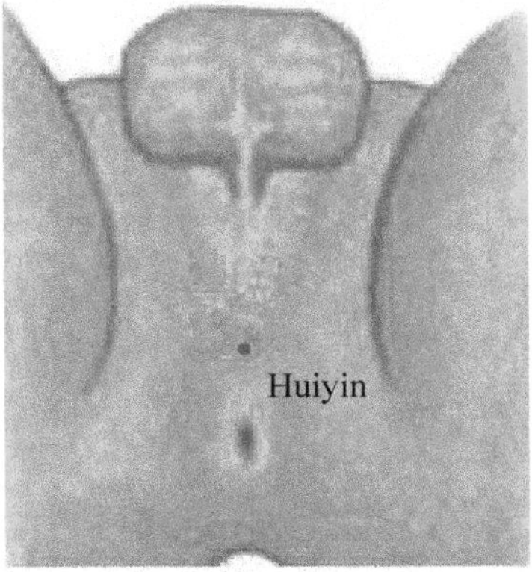

Fig. 4-33

图书在版编目（CIP）数据

健身祛病的夫妻互助按摩法 ：英文 / 张树林编著. -- 北京 ：
新世界出版社，2014.8
ISBN 978-7-5104-4398-5

Ⅰ. ①健… Ⅱ. ①张… Ⅲ. ①按摩疗法（中医）—英文
Ⅳ. ①R244.1

中国版本图书馆 CIP 数据核字（2014）第 186744 号

Healthcare Massage for Your Partner
健身祛病的夫妻互助按摩法

编 著 者：张树林
翻　　译：吴雪君　王　秒　徐　晖
英文审定：Anja Matthey de I'Etang
责任编辑：张建平
封面设计：张　薇
责任印制：李一鸣　黄厚清
出版发行：新世界出版社
社　　址：北京西城区百万庄大街24号（100037）
发行部：(010) 6899 5968　(010) 6899 8705（传真）
总编室：(010) 6899 5424　(010) 6832 6679（传真）
http://www.nwp.cn
http://www.newworld-press.com
版权部：+8610 6899 6306
版权部电子信箱：frank@nwp.com.cn
印刷：北京京华虎彩印刷有限公司
经销：新华书店
开本：787×1092　1/32
字数：190千字　　印张：8
版次：2014年8月第1版　2014年8月北京第1次印刷
书号：ISBN 978-5104-4398-5
定价：68.00元